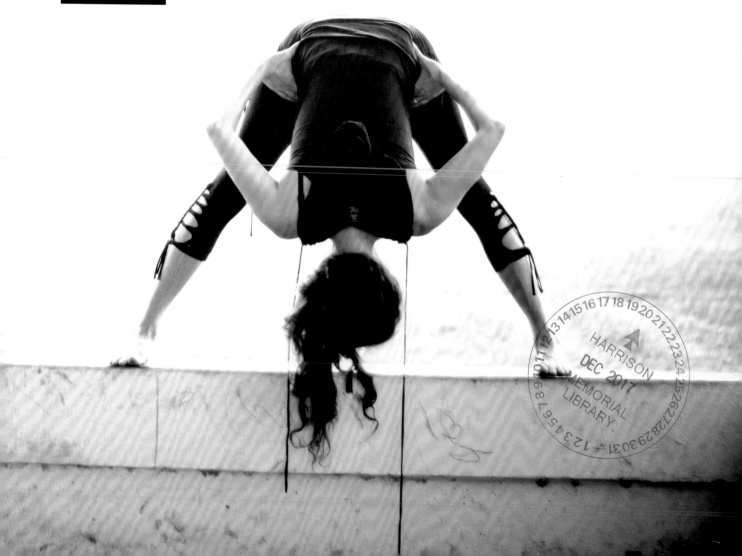

" YOGA TEACHES US
TO CURE WHAT NEED NOT
BE ENDURED AND ENDURE
WHAT CANNOT BE CURED"

B.K.S. IYENGAR

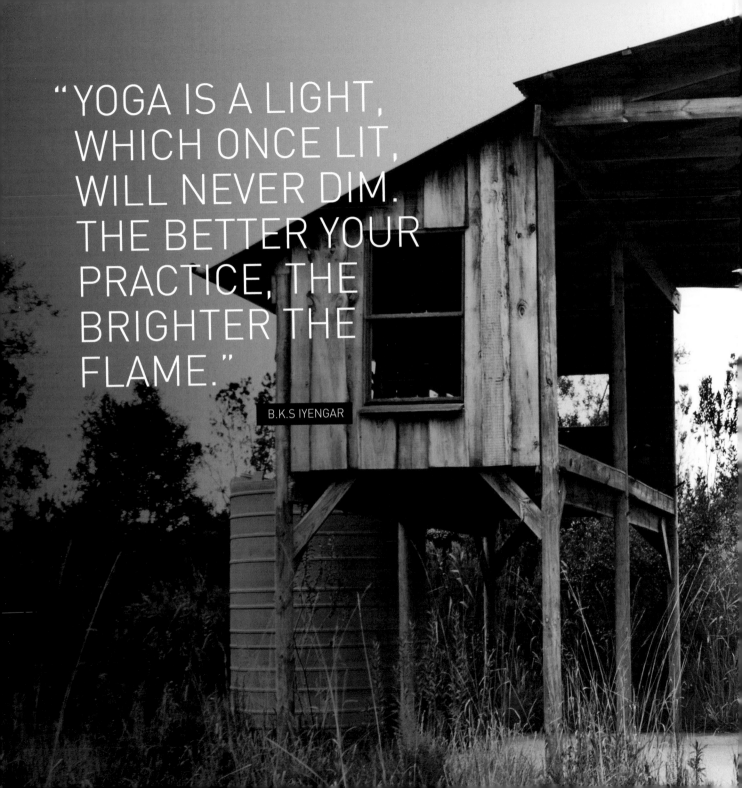

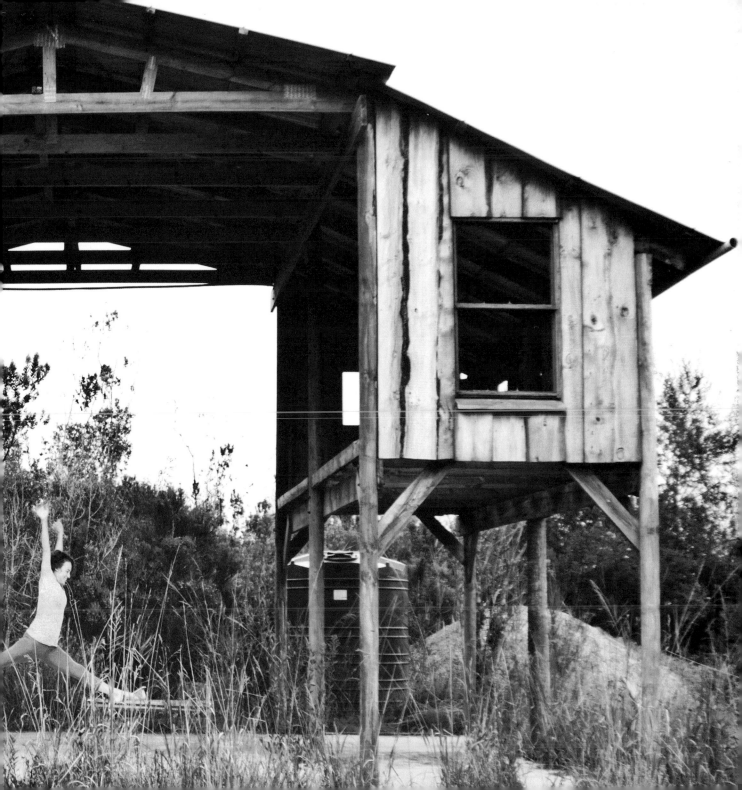

"BY EMBRACING YOUR MOTHER WOUND AS YOUR YOGA, YOU TRANSFORM WHAT HAS BEEN A HINDRANCE IN YOUR LIFE INTO A TEACHER OF THE HEART."

PHILLIP MOFFITT

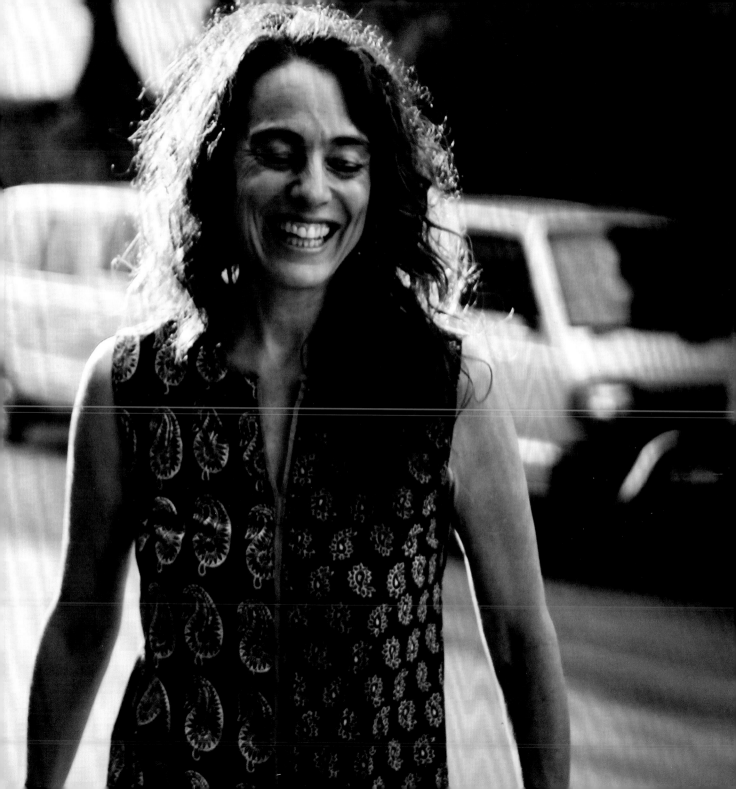

Disclaimer: Rachel Zinman is not a medical doctor. This book is not intended as a substitute for the medical advice of physicians. The reader should regularly consult a physician in matters relating to his/her health including the advisability of practicing yoga, and particularly with respect to any symptoms that may require diagnosis or medical attention.

Paperback ISBN: 978-1-939681-76-8
eBook ISBN: 978-1-939681-77-5

Library of Congress Cataloging-in-Publication Data

Names: Zinman, Rachel, author.
Title: Yoga for diabetes : how to manage your health with yoga and ayurveda / Rachel Zinman.
Description: Rhinebeck, New York : Monkfish Book Publishing Company, [2017]
Identifiers: LCCN 2017008601 | ISBN 9781939681768 (pbk. : alk. paper)
Subjects: LCSH: Diabetes--Alternative treatment--Popular works. | Hatha yoga--Therapeutic use. | Medicine, Ayurvedic. | Self-care, Health--Popular works.
Classification: LCC RC661.A47 Z56 2017 | DDC 616.4/62062--dc23
LC record available at https://lccn.loc.gov/2017008601

Image Credits:
David Young - Front Cover, Back Cover, p.136, 141, 160-161, 162, 165, 166, 169, 170, 173, 174, 177, 178, 181, 182, 185, 186, 189, 190, 193, 194, 196-197, 198, 201, 202, 205, 206, 209, 210, 213, 214, 217, 218, 221, 222, 225, 226, 229, 230, 233, 234, 237, 238, 240-241, 242, 245, 246, 249, 250, 253-254, 257, 258, 261, 262, 265, 266, 269, 270, 273, 274, 277, 278, 281, 282, 285, 286, 291-300.
Nora Wendel p.1, 2-3, 4-5, 6, 7, 8, 11, 12, 18, 19, 27, 62, 67, 69, 75, 77, 115, 117, 119, 124, 134, 139, 144, 151, 153, 310 www.norawendel.com
Heather Elton p.75 model   www.eltonyoga.com
Rachel Hull Ayurvedic Questionnaire p.156-157

Graphic design by Maraya Rodostianos
Editing by Kris Emery
Printed in China

Monkfish Book Publishing Company
22 East Market Street, Suite 304
Rhinebeck, NY 12572
(845) 876-4861
www.monkfishpublishing.com

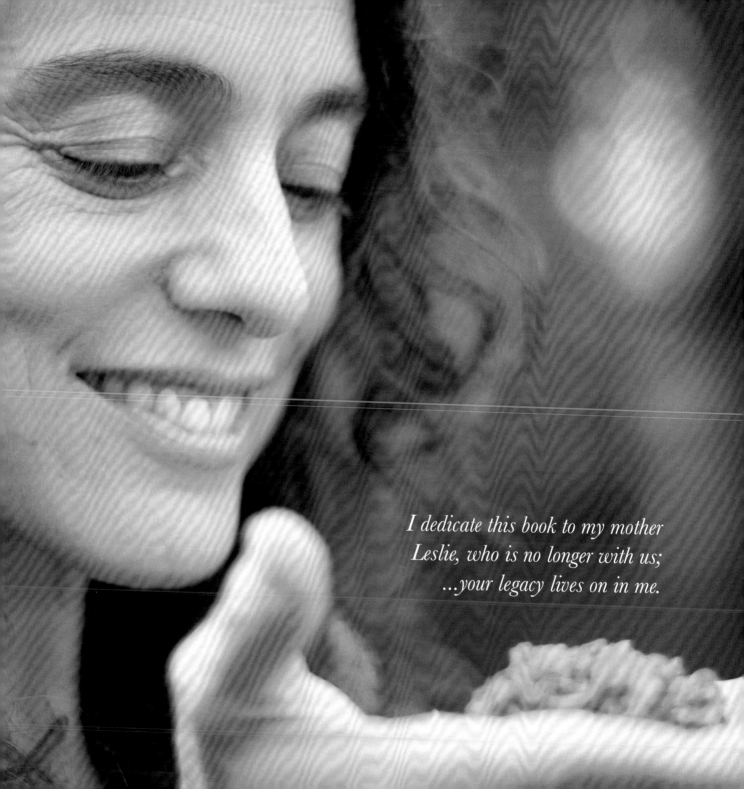

I dedicate this book to my mother
Leslie, who is no longer with us;
...your legacy lives on in me.

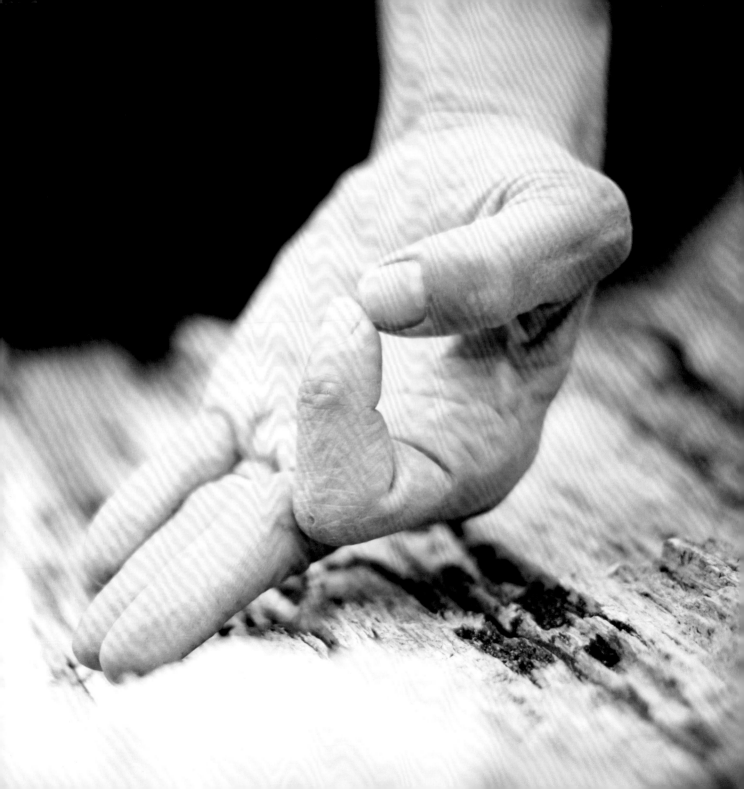

Contents

contents continued...

contents continued...

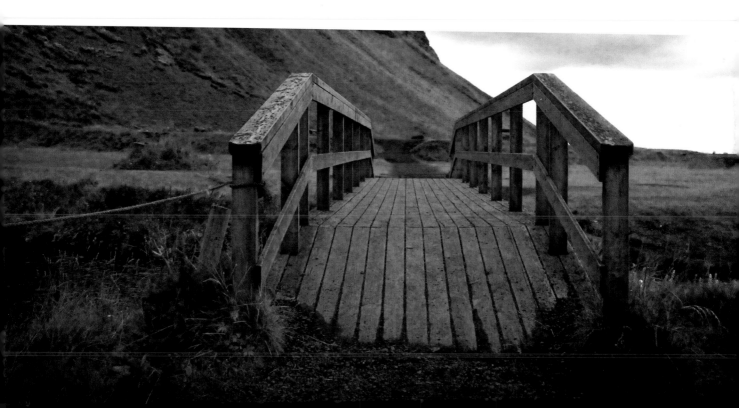

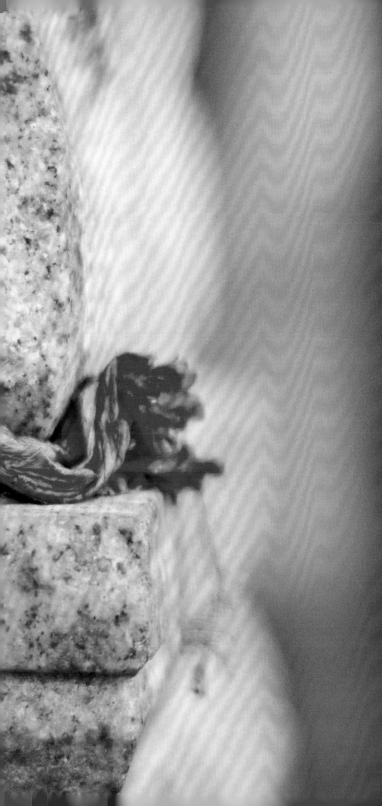

| Testimonials

"Our teacher Krishnamacharya was a master physician as well as yoga master. He perfected the skill of adapting yoga to individual needs including healing illness. Rachel has studied yoga diligently, practiced and overcome illness in her personal life. I urge you to read this book and find out how easy it is to implement a powerful healing yoga practice in your life."

~ **Mark Whitwell, author of** *Yoga of Heart* **and** *The Promise*
  heartofyoga.com

"I have known Rachel since she came to teach for me at Be Yoga in Manhattan in 2000. A passionate student, it wasn't long before she became an integral member of my team. Her dedication and devotion to yoga showed up in every aspect of her life. But there were also challenges. Rachel and I worked together over years to help her manage her overall health and wellbeing. I am so pleased that she has brought to life the many things I shared with her in how to approach yoga for the individual. No matter what type of diabetes you have, knowing how to meet your needs through the various practices of posture, breath and meditation can make a world of difference. I highly recommend this book for anyone wanting to manage their health and experience the profound healing nature of yoga. Rachel truly shares from her heart."

~ **Alan Finger, Ishta Yoga founder**
  ishtayoga.com

"Your story is heart-wrenching. Thank you for giving everyone the gift of your sharing, honesty, vulnerability. You are so amazing, so brave, so courageous. What you are giving is a priceless gift, and not just to diabetics, but to anyone grappling with a chronic health condition. I love how Yoga for Diabetes gains momentum into the deepest and most complex issues related to diabetes and then simplifies this information and makes it accessible to everyone no matter what stage they're in."

~ **Lisa Fitzpatrick, bestselling author & owner of Sacred Women's Business**
  lisafitzpatrick.com.au

"Rachel's passion for both yoga and her wellbeing as a person with diabetes is what makes this book come alive. It reminds me how much yoga changed my own life as a person with diabetes. She is a real person who faces the challenges we all face with diabetes, but yoga lit a light in her that makes the burden of type 1 diabetes so much lighter. And she's sharing that light with her readers. If you're looking for the inspiration to feel more connected and appreciative of your body, and what it's capable of, rather than feeling defeated and frustrated, Rachel and her yoga education will support you in that journey!"

~ Ginger Vieira, author & editorial director
diabetesdaily.com

"Rachel Zinman is a gifted writer. Becoming a diabetic created a crisis in her life, a journey that she writes about with great vulnerability. Instead of succumbing to despair, Rachel has committed herself to sharing her experiences of healing through this book, online and in workshops. In Yoga for Diabetes, Rachel weaves together all she has learned in 30 years of yoga practice with newfound knowledge and skills. She presents these in a thoroughly interesting and available way that is suitable for an audience ranging from beginners to yoga teachers, and other health practitioners. This is a lifestyle book for people with diabetes. Yoga for Diabetes offers information on how to support one's health in the most holistic way. In simple terms, Rachel explains the Ayurvedic approach to managing diabetes with diet, breathing exercises, physical yoga and meditation. These complement a protocol of medication, diet and exercise, and offer the best opportunity for a person living with diabetes to enjoy a healthy, balanced life. No matter what stresses life throws up."

~ Eve Grzybowski, founder of Sydney Yoga Centre
eveyoga.com

"With great compassion and clarity, Rachel Zinman introduces people with diabetes to the benefits of yoga, meditation and Ayurveda, specific to each individual's nature. Rachel's lifelong passion for yoga, melded with her coming to terms with a diagnosis of type 1 diabetes as an adult, provides a profound service to those of us with diabetes. Yes, we must take our meds (including exogenous insulin for those of us with type 1 diabetes) and follow our treatment protocols, but we can also find some peace and space amidst the challenge of diabetes. Rachel shows us how."

~ Melitta Rorty, yoga practitioner and blogger on adult-onset type 1 diabetes
adultt1diabetes.blogspot.com

"For many people, yoga provides a way to stay fit, find balance in their lives on and off the mat, and (hopefully) connect with themselves on the deepest level. For others, it's a mere fad that they've sampled and abandoned when the next 'new' thing came along. Rachel Zinman, on the other hand, has devoted her life to the study and practice not only of yoga but of Ayurveda, the ancient Indian 'science of life,' healing techniques that go way beyond any Western definition of medicine. It was only natural that when, despite a life of extraordinarily healthy practice and diet, Rachel was diagnosed with type 1 diabetes, she would turn to yoga and Ayurveda for tools to supplement insulin injections and other modern ways of treating her disease. This book offers a unique lens not only into how yoga and Ayurveda can help diabetics of all types live more easily with this disease, but how even the sources and manifestations of diabetes arise from the type of person we each are and the lifestyle choices we have made. Throughout, Rachel's artful prose and compelling honesty make this a page-turner even for those never touched by diabetes. Rachel writes with clarity, candour and authenticity that will inspire anyone's life with diabetes, and may well prod others to seek out yoga and/or Ayurveda in coping with other diseases. It's clear from the first sentence that she's one of us!"

~ Lois Nesbitt Ph.D., E-RYT, author of *Hip Op: Beyond Recovery!*
loisnesbittyoga.com

Acknowledgments

First off, I want to thank my parents, Mary and David Zinman. I feel they instilled in me such a strong appreciation for creativity, the arts and being myself. I have always felt them nearby, no matter where I am in the world. I respect and admire them both immensely and couldn't have asked for better role models.

I also thank my partner John, who in the last five years has been a rock of support. It's because of him and the wonderful teachings that he shares that I have been able to view my condition as something I have rather than something I am. His ability to make me laugh, his firmness of conviction, and his delight in life and creation are such an inspiration to me. Every day I am blown away that we met and how delightful the journey is with him.

My son Jacob has also played a huge part in bringing me to where I am today. I never imagined I'd have a child and when I did it wasn't anything I could have expected. Being a mother literally grew me up and at the same time allowed me to be a child again. To foster another's growth and creativity, while setting them free, another milestone. Now that my son is grown, I admire his caring nature. He has stood by me, supported me and made the journey with this condition just that little bit easier.

I'd like to thank my ex-husband Nicholas, who spent years supporting my passion for creative expression. As a team, we sang, danced, wrote, travelled and parented, and even though our time together came to an end, I will be forever grateful for all the encouragement he gave me to write my story, for all the tears we shed and all the dreams we explored.

Beyond my close family, I wish to acknowledge the friends in my life who have encouraged me to express my truth. To my friend Vatika Gow, who walked with me through country lanes, while listening to my ups and downs. To my friend Louisa Sear, who started me on my yoga journey and has continued to support me to this day. To my mentor and teacher Alan Finger, who initiated me into the science of Ayurveda, the joys of Tantra and its wonderful tools of mantra and yantra. Many of the tools and practices in the book come from my studies with Alan. And to all my students, without whom I wouldn't be teaching and sharing. Your enthusiasm for yoga has made it all worthwhile.

The idea for the book and its creation wouldn't be possible without the kind support of some really special people. I'd like to thank Shaz Rhodes. She dreamed up the idea, gave me a visual download and now it's a book in your hands. A huge thank you to Jacinta McEwan, Lisa Fitzpatrick, Ginger Vieira and Kimmana Nichols for feedback on the various chapters. I'd like to thank David Young, Maraya Rodostianos and Kris Emery for putting the whole book together in its present form.

A huge thank you to my support team during our photoshoots, Noriko Wrencher, Jody Vassallo, Shaz Rhodes, Kavi Jarrot, Marie Baker, Meredith Bask and Lyn Ruming, Lisa and Robert Bleakley and Naren King from the Crystal Castle for providing stunning locations. I couldn't have done it without you. I'd also like to thank Susi Plesser from Divine Goddess Yoga Products for donating all the yoga clothes for our shoot. And a big thank you to Nora Wendel for offering her beautiful photos to complete the package.

I'd also like to acknowledge the generous support of the businesses here in my home town of Mullumbimby, New South Wales. To the team at Mullum Herbals, Jacinta, Elvian, Val and the gang. Your herbal remedies, Ayurvedic advice, and availability and experience has helped me time and time again, from consults to pick-me-ups to a hug when I needed it. I can't recommend these guys highly enough.

To my dear friend Michael Collis, who has worked his magic with acupuncture on me since I was 21. Michael taught me how to live a healthy lifestyle, rooted for me when the chips were down and has been a lifeline through this challenging journey.

I also want to acknowledge the generous support of The Art of Healing magazine, one of the only health and wellbeing magazines I trust to deliver accurate information on how to sustain a lifestyle using holistic methods.

A special thank you to Leann Harris from Delphi Diabetes Coaching and Corey Johnson from Zenflow for winning our business sponsorship award. You can find out more about their wonderful businesses in the resource section.

Thank you to Linda Balon Stein from Zosimos Botanicals, who I've known since I was seven years old. I am so grateful for Linda's support in enabling me to produce this book and love how her natural cosmetic range is designed for people just like me who are super sensitive to chemicals.

Thank you to Yoga Trail for being the premier network promoting yoga teachers worldwide, for getting behind this project and spreading the word. And a big thank you to Yoga Australia for being a credible body of information for yoga teachers and therapists in Australia.

I'd like to thank my team of diabetes sisters, Cynthia Zuber, Melitta Rorty, Michelle Sorenson, Karen Rose Tank, Riva Greenberg, Karen Eivers, Leora Krowitz, Daniele Hargenrader, Marina Tsaplina, Asha Brown, Dr Jody Stanislaw, Leann Harris, Anna Hruby, Danidoo Butterfly, Carolyn Miller, Bonnie Sher, Helen Edwards and Ginger Vieira. Your feedback support and genuine enthusiasm has made it so much easier for me to get the word out there in the diabetes online community.

And to all the people who donated generously to the crowdfunding campaign, Yoga Synergy, Paul Druzinsky, Chris Barret, Karen Boren Gerstenberger, Jeanette Darbyshire, Simone and Mal Odgers, Rachel Hull, Patricia Walters, Snehy Gupta, Miriam Katz, Allan Rosen, Margaret Cohen, Amir and Nirupa Hoffman, Oscar Sellerach and Caroline Cowley, Victoria Gilbert Duca, Andrew Canet, Lisa Peers, Claudia Scheurer, Anna Hruby, Maz Jeffreys, Laura Fernandez Moso, Michael Collis, Mullum Herbals, Alka Franco, Romina DiFederico, Felicity Slee, Adam Furnell and Belinda Philp, Jen Jones-Wilton, Catherina Anne Doyle, Ronit Robbaz, Twee Merrigan, Deborah Hennessey, Gaby Aschwanden, Jodi Mann, Stephen Brookes, Piari Leibo, Hiroshi Funakoshi, Enrico John, Delsie Dunn, Susan Reinhart, Di Tucker-Benzaquen, Patrizia Strub-Wohlwend, Sabina Dods, Nadja Warner, Shari Reiman, David Fogarty, Anna Marti, Amber Spear, Natalie Snooke, Aaron Cohen, Lis Wallace, Jacob Zinman-Jeanes, Tamara Graham, Sharon M Kenny, Nora Wendel, Mona Anand, Sally Brown, Riana Begg, Michele Dalle-Nogare, Maz Jefferys, Naomi Gregory, Emil Wendel and Anouk, Priya Link, Anna Hruby, Toby Strogatz, Kumiko Mack, Lainie Jenkins, Julie Ann Martin, Julian Yudelson, Rainer Heigl, Christine Thompson, Bob & Bev Murphy, Lorenzo Ammendola, Linda Balon Stein, Sali Mcintyre, Anna Moskvina and Bodaniel Jeanes. Thank you all.

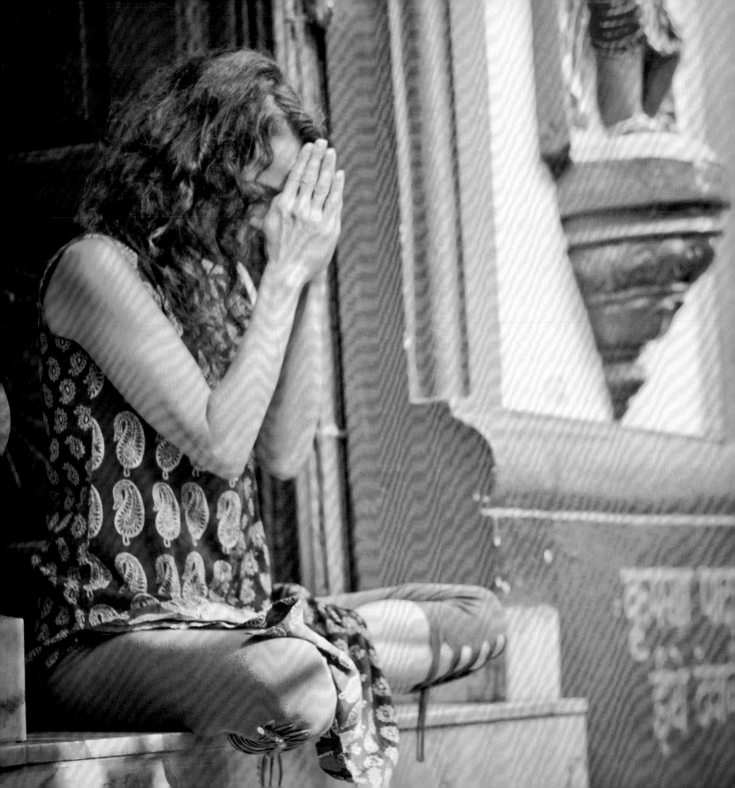

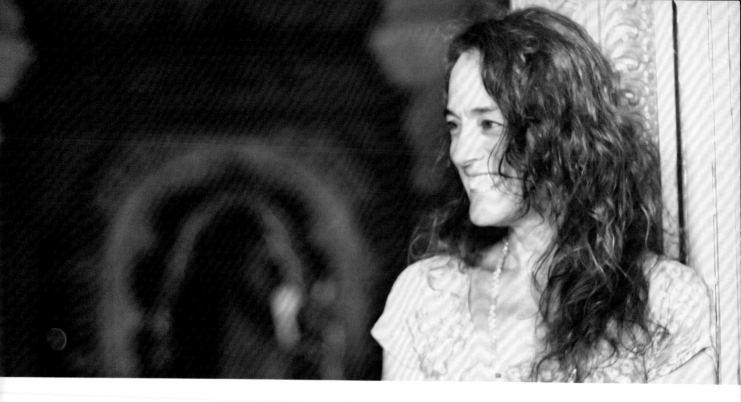

| Why diabetes? Why me?

If you've started practicing and are curious about how yoga can support you in your diabetes care, let me assure you, you're in the right place.

I've met some people with type 1 diabetes who took up yoga post-diagnosis and plenty of type 2s who practice regularly. But it's rarer to meet a yogi who developed type 1 as an adult. That's exactly what happened to me. It took six years for me to accept my diagnosis of type 1 diabetes and a "lifetime" to find a story I felt passionate enough to write. Despite how long I took to come to terms with diabetes, I have nothing but gratitude for what's happened to me. I'm now excited to share all the practices that can help you enjoy the benefits yoga brings. But first, here's my story:

I'd always been obsessive about my body. I'd long been afraid that I'd get some disease or other. Most likely this is because my mother died when I was 11. She had a stroke first and then passed away during an operation to remove a brain tumor. Coincidentally her mother, my grandmother also had a brain tumor, but she survived and lived well into her 80s. My mother died just one month after her 40th birthday.

Even though I'd convinced myself I would suffer some disease, I never really focused on the fact that diabetes ran in my family. I remember my grandmother was diagnosed with it late in life, a complication from being paralyzed on her right side which led to a sedentary lifestyle. When I was diagnosed at 42, both of my maternal aunts clamored to tell me that my great-grandfather had had diabetes as well before there was insulin, and my great-uncle had been on insulin.

My diagnosis was sudden, but I didn't have many symptoms. It came through a random blood test. I'd been a bit fatigued, but I'd put it down to adrenal burnout. I'd been getting dizzy whenever I ate dates. In fact, I was feeling overwhelmed by sugary foods in general, but nothing I couldn't handle, so I thought. I'd practiced yoga most of my life and had been seeing naturopaths and chiropractors since I was 19. I remember my first foray into eating 'clean' was with the candida diet. While everyone else was downing candy bars, I was drinking drops of tea tree oil and avoiding dairy, wheat and sugar. But like any normal 20-something, I couldn't stay on that diet forever. Eventually my life settled into normal. I got married, had a baby, and did yoga to stay fit. I ended up teaching and that was that.

In those days, yoga wasn't the fitness craze it is today. It was esoteric and spiritual. My body has always been sensitive and the yoga amped up that sensitivity. I was into Ashtanga yoga, which is an athletic style. Yet while it opened up my body, it also released a lot of toxins. I don't think I was more toxic than anybody else per se, but because I'd never processed my mother's death, there was generalized unease and uncertainty in my body, which created unconscious stress. Before I was serious about yoga, I was a promising dancer and choreographer, but I never felt quite up to par. I was constantly getting distracted by one boy or another and could never commit fully to the craft. In the end, I chose a relationship over dance. And then, when I became bored out of my mind, I dove headlong into yoga.

That's when everything shifted. I saw yoga as the ultimate way to perfect the body--my free pass from insecurity to security. After 10 years of consistent yoga and meditation practice, I moved my family from Byron Bay, Australia to New York City. Without intending to, I met my teacher Alan Finger, a lovely Buddha-like man who'd been doing yoga since he was 15 and teaching for most of his life. He seemed to know me better than I knew myself and taught techniques I'd never seen or heard of before. In his presence, my restless mind went still. I was lucky enough to teach for him at his school and help train other teachers. And even though I had a young son, a stepson and a husband at home, I thrived on the busyness of my life. I worked from dawn till late at night, forgetting to eat or rest. I absolutely loved teaching and practicing and learning as much as I could about yoga. It was a lifeline, a way to tranquillize the insecurities and fears from my younger years. Even though I could feel the stress building from my relentless schedule, I somehow didn't care.

Then 9/11 happened.

That day was terrible, terrible for everyone.

I was in Manhattan waiting for Alan to teach his yoga class when the planes hit the trade towers. As soon as I realized what had happened, I felt like I'd been shot in the chest, my legs buckling underneath me. After a few minutes, I had to get out of there. My son and stepson were at school a few blocks away from the yoga studio and I wanted to be with them. Dazed and feeling sick to my stomach, I walked out onto the street. It was quiet; ghost-like. People with ashen faces walked beside me. The sky was a crisp blue and I wondered how everyone could keep on going.

By the time I arrived at the school, I was feeling faint. I wanted someone to hold me and look after me, but I wasn't the only one in shock. I had to pull myself together. It was a relief to have both boys with me. The only way home to Brooklyn was to walk across the 59th Street Bridge. I could feel fear stuck in my throat, dry and hard. Gripping my sons' hands, we walked.

Nearly seven hours after the towers had fallen, I fell into my husband's arms, but it was no consolation for the shock that numbed my body. I couldn't eat, couldn't even think because my whole world had turned upside down.

Emotionally and physically, I never recovered from that day. And although I can't specifically pinpoint my diabetes onset, I started experiencing a lot of strange physical symptoms about a year later. Tingling up and down my body, difficulty concentrating, insomnia, a feeling of being overly expanded, frequent urination, hives and skin rashes, racing heartbeat, difficulty with my digestion and many more symptoms that turned my life into a living hell.

I spent most of my time trying to work out what wouldn't trigger me, restricting my diet and my activities, but all the while I had to make money and keep teaching yoga.

The first clue that it might be something to do with my pancreas was on holiday in England. I went to a day clinic because I was peeing every few minutes and I thought I had the start of a UTI. The nurse asked me if I'd ever had a blood sugar test and pricked my finger. I still remember the reading on the meter: 5.5. She said it was normal and I was sent on my way with a sachet to alkalize my urine.

Eventually, I left America with my family and moved back to our home in Byron Bay, Australia. Once there, I started treatments with an acupuncturist who kept pointing out that my symptoms were remarkably similar to those of someone who has diabetes. I kept getting my fasting levels checked, but nothing seemed out of the ordinary so I still didn't

I'll never forget that moment of diagnosis and how my breath caught in my chest. I felt like I was drowning...

pick up that there was a problem until...the day my husband interrupted my morning yoga practice to inform me that the doctor had discovered 'something bad' in my blood work.

What followed was a horrendous visit to the doctor where I was told that my A1c was slightly elevated and that I had diabetes. He shoved a few pamphlets in my direction and hustled me out of the room with advice to Google 'diabetes' and buy a glucometer so I could test my blood glucose levels. He intimated that it would take years to cure myself. I'll never forget that moment of diagnosis and how my breath caught in my chest. I felt like I was drowning. Angry and confused, I was sure I'd done something wrong. It reminded me of how I felt when my mother died. I wanted to run away but there was nowhere to hide. The feeling of terror and hopelessness was palpable. I kept playing his words over and over in my head, asking myself, where did I go wrong? Surely this was all a big mistake.

Thankfully, this doctor was not my endocrinologist, whom I saw a few days later. The endo painted a much more palatable picture of the slow onset of my disease and outlined the likely steps I might need to take as the disease progressed. His words definitely reassured me but I was still in shock. How could a yoga teacher and health-conscious person like me get diabetes? It would take me years to stop blaming myself.

At first I told myself that I didn't actually have diabetes and that somehow both doctors had made a mistake. I decided to take matters into my own hands and saw an ayurvedic doctor in India. After reading my pulse, she told me that the type of diabetes I had was very hard to cure but not impossible and gave me a long list of foods and herbs with the advice to eat eight small meals a day. I followed her advice religiously for two years until eventually, not seeing much improvement, I tried Japanese acupuncture.

The acupuncturist agreed with me that I couldn't have diabetes. Instead my symptoms were indicative that my spleen wasn't functioning well. He assured me that with weekly sessions and herbal formulas my blood sugar levels which were still slightly elevated would return to normal. Although my levels stabilized they did not improve enough for me to feel that it was working. My next step was to visit a nutritionist and naturopath who specialized in healing gut disorders. She was also adamant that I didn't have diabetes. She surmised that my high blood sugar was caused by a parasitic infection that I'd picked up on my travels to East Asia. I was so relieved after seeing her that I phoned my parents to tell them the good news. A few weeks later, while visiting them, I overheard them telling friends, "it's not diabetes anymore, Rachel just has a parasite."

Besides enrolling my parents in my ongoing ideas about what I did or didn't have, I took pills, swallowed concoctions, tried to heal my microbiome and prayed! Three months later my blood sugar levels were higher than ever.

As a last resort I was able to score an appointment with a famous Ayurvedic doctor who told me that what I really was suffering from was EMF (Electro Magnetic Frequency) poisoning and that his super special licorice cream and homeopathic drops would do the trick. After lathering myself in creams for 6 months and spending thousands of dollars for his magic potions I was no better.

By now, nearly six years on from my diagnosis, I was miserable, frustrated and at my wits end. At this point my doctor recommended insulin to get my levels under control.

I remember thinking that there was no way I would ever take medication. I was terrified that I would react to the insulin in some way and get even sicker. I kept telling myself, tomorrow things will get better, I'll wake up with a normal blood sugar level and this nightmare will end.

But it didn't.

After dragging myself up and down hills and restricting my diet to almost nothing I began to notice a constant tingling in my hands and feet. The doctor insisted I see a neurologist. I was so adept at making excuses that

I told him not to worry and that it was probably a B12 deficiency. But the neurologist confirmed otherwise. I had the beginning of neuropathy and I definitely had diabetes. He gave me a stern warning to get my levels down or face permanent nerve damage.

That's when I hit rock bottom. I had no idea how I could have let things get so out of control. As a yoga teacher I was supposed to lead by example and here I was, in the pit of denial, dealing with blood sugar levels that were so high I should have been in a hospital.

I finally admitted to myself that my body wasn't able to produce enough insulin anymore and that no matter what I thought, or what kind of healer I thought could cure me it was time for me to listen to my doctor, to start taking insulin and to accept my diagnosis.

When I'm on the mat, breathing or sitting quietly, there's no me, mine or I. I am not the disease; I have a disease.

Starting anything new and changing habits isn't easy. All my habits with food, exercise and sleep were let go with reluctance. Every time I tried to break a pattern, I had to stop and ask myself, "What's more important? Eating what I want, when I want, or living a full, energetic and productive life?"

Family and friends often comment on how disciplined I am and how they could never do it. In the early days when I started managing my disease through diet and exercise, I never told them how hard it was to sit and watch everybody eat pizza and chocolate mousse, while I ate a spinach omelet with no dessert.

Now I tell it like it is. This disease sucks! And if it weren't for my daily yoga and meditation practice, I don't think I'd cope. I've experienced depression, lethargy, hopelessness, fear and anger. But in spite of those very real emotions, I do accept what's happened to me.

Just shortly after diagnosis, I visited a friend whose son had diabetes. Diagnosed at eight years old, he showed me how to use my newly acquired glucometer then casually pulled up his shirt and inserted a needle into his belly. He seemed so nonchalant when he spoke about the disease, sharing that it was a 24/7 affair, no days off. Sad but true.

The disease seemed almost external to him. Like a visitor he had to entertain.

It reminded me of how I feel when I practice yoga. When I'm on the mat, breathing or sitting quietly, there's no me, mine or I. I am not the disease; I have a disease.

Separating who we are from what we have is one of the first steps in depersonalizing ourselves from our illness. It's also a meaningful aspect of yoga. In traditional teachings, yoga is seen as a separation from all the beliefs we have about ourselves. And there's no bigger belief than we are our bodies. It's simple logic. If the body doesn't feel good, we don't feel good.

What does yoga offer us?

A simple break from the intensity of all that the body throws at us.

The good feelings that come after a yoga class not only arise from the act of stretching and massaging all the muscles and organs, but a brief respite from our need to buy into all those beliefs about our bodies. I like to think of it as being on holiday; you're sitting on a beach somewhere admiring the view, feeling happy and at peace, and in that moment you're not thinking about your disease. You're content. Where did all the worries go? Nowhere. You just stopped identifying with them.

In a nutshell, that's what happens during a yoga practice. And the more we can get a break from our identification with the thoughts about our disease, the more the nervous system relaxes and the more easily we can manage our health.

In all the literature I have read or information I have heard about autoimmune conditions, there is a consensus that heredity and environmental causes are just two-thirds of the total picture. Stress and our inability to handle it is the third component. If we can reduce our stress, the immune system catches a break and we can slow the progression of our condition, force it into remission or at the very least manage it with fewer complications.

I wish I could say I have high hopes for a cure for type 1 diabetes. But to be honest, I don't. I'm not fatalistic about it either though. It's just that after working like a dog for years to cure myself with everything including Ayurveda, acupuncture, herbs, diet and homeopathic medicine, all I managed to do was slow its progression. I still have had to go on insulin and deal with nerve damage as well as thyroid and pituitary issues.

It hasn't been easy facing my situation when I'd spent most of my life thinking yoga was a cure-all. It's been a rude awakening having to completely reevaluate the role that yoga plays, not only in my life but in the life of anyone with an incurable disease. In reality, what does yoga do? What is its purpose? And how can it be used to manage disease?

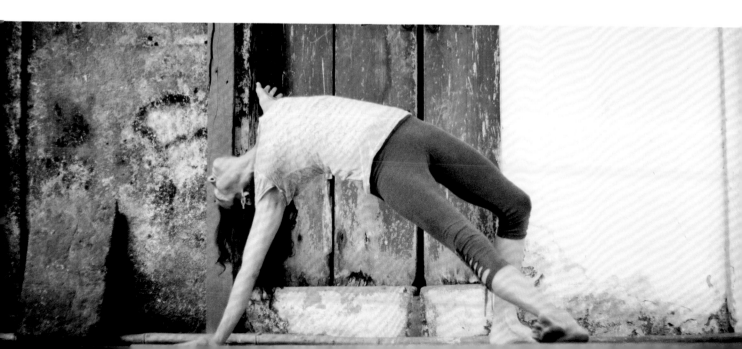

| The Purpose of YOGA

Helping you to understand the role of yoga in managing disease is the purpose and subject of this book. Here, I present the practices, lifestyle changes and systems of thought that enable me to face this condition each and every day with a positive outlook, and that I hope will be life-changing for you too. I feel incredibly lucky to have been diagnosed at a time where insulin therapy is relatively painless and conveniently administered. The technologies around glucose control, the latest research on diet and all the other factors that contribute to saving lives each and every day are mind-blowing. Coming out of denial and discovering a whole community online where people are sharing not only their struggles but their triumphs is uplifting; I no longer feel like I'm doing this on my own.

Throughout my life, I have always wanted to help others, but simultaneously found it difficult to take responsibility for helping myself. Taking up a yoga practice, eating wholesome and nurturing foods, living life with devotion and reverence are just some of the ways I consciously give back to myself on a day-to-day basis. My life as a yogi is not a fad. And having a disease like diabetes, I can't afford to be part of a trend anyway. That's why I feel strongly that the simplicity and discipline of yoga, plus the lifestyle guidelines from Ayurveda are the perfect starting point no matter what type of diabetes you have. The postural sequences, breathing and meditation techniques, thoughts on yoga and its deeper meaning, and the Ayurvedic lifestyle suggestions are there to support you in facing some of the challenges that come with the disease. And top of that list, of course, are stress and burnout.

I am confident that like me you will discover that yoga is a life-changing and life-enhancing system. And a great friend and companion that will hold your hand through all the ups and downs you are bound to experience.

With great respect,

Rachel

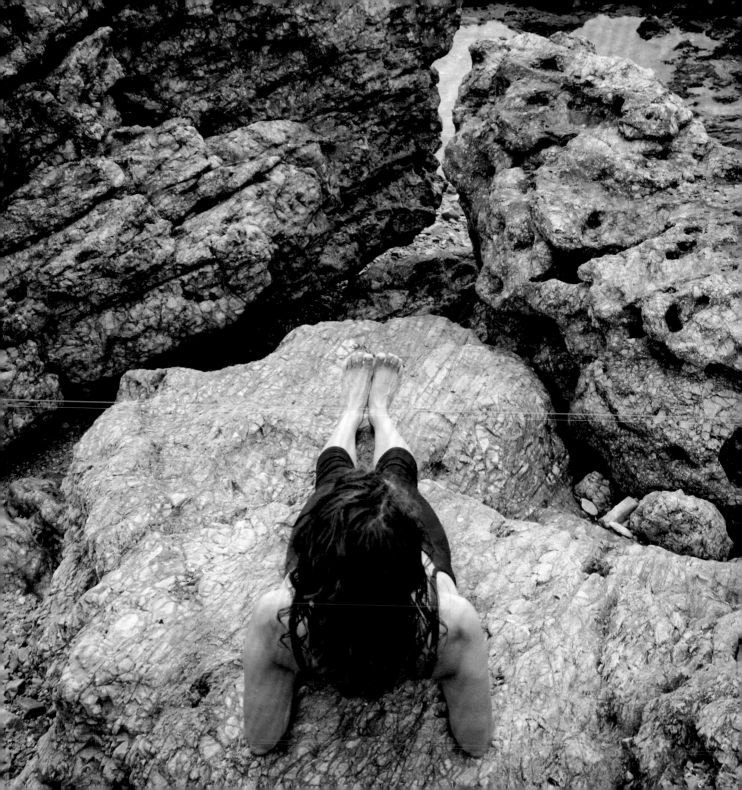

CHAPTER ONE
A LIFESTYLE AND A SCIENCE

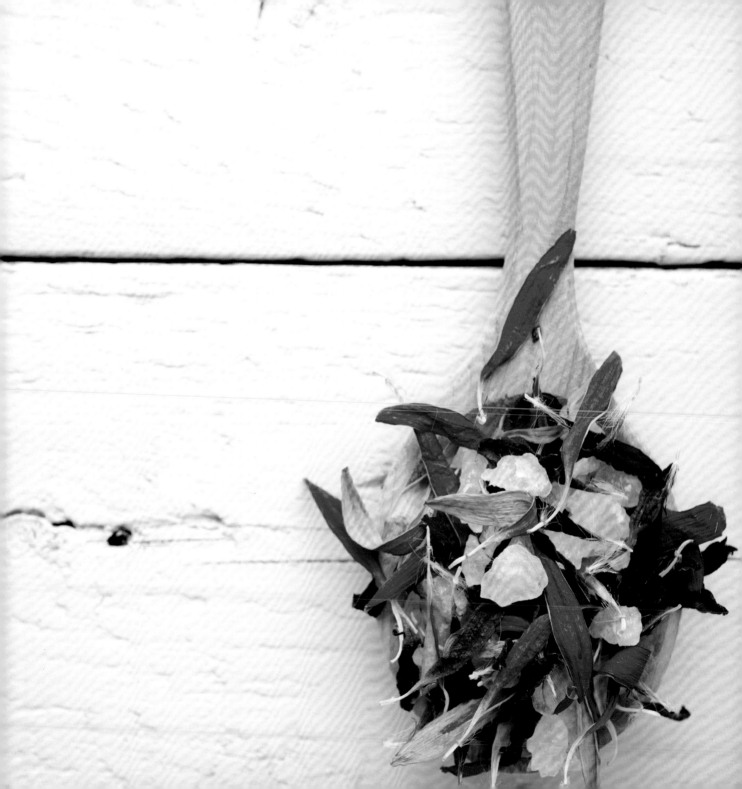

| What type of diabetes do I have?

You've been diagnosed with either type 1, type 2, type 1 LADA, gestational diabetes, MODY or perhaps you're a parent reading this on behalf of your child who has been diagnosed with juvenile diabetes. There is a ton of literature, books and resources out there about the type of disease you have, and with those come the various medications, lifestyle and dietary guidelines.

But did you know that the ancient science of Ayurveda has been working with diabetes for 4,000 years since Vedic times? The Vedas, the oldest scriptures in Hinduism, were composed between 1750–500 BCE. Back then, the disease was called prameha which means major disease, as almost every part of the body and every cell is affected by diabetes.

Prameha was then divided into two subcategories:

1. **Apatharpana uthaja prameha** describing the 'lean' diabetic.
2. **Santharpana uthaja prameha** relating to the diabetic who was overweight.

The fancy Sanskrit names are irrelevant to us today but it's interesting to note that, just like our current understanding of the causes of diabetes, Ayurveda distinguishes between the two as follows:

1. **Sahaja prameha** - genetic.
2. **Apathyanimittaja prameha** - due to excess.

From there, Ayurveda sees the disease as manifesting in the three different Ayurvedic constitutions.

But let's back up a bit... because to understand which constitution you have and how that relates to your type of diabetes, you'll need the background story.

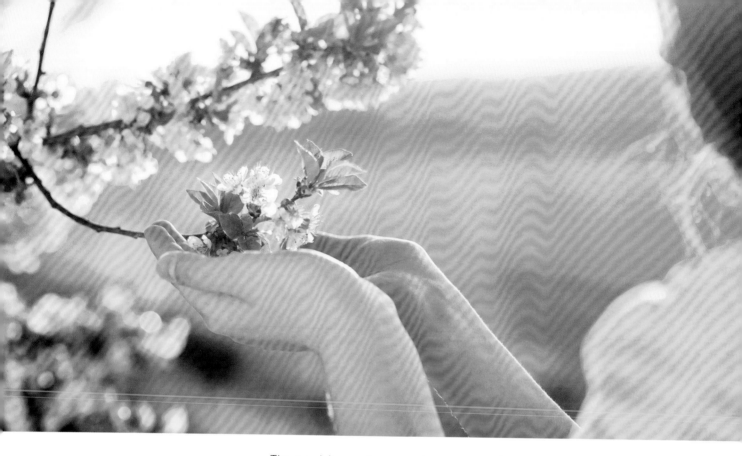

The word Ayurveda comes from two words: ayus and veda. Ayus means life; 'life' being your body, mind, senses and associated organs. Veda means science. So Ayurveda literally means 'the science of life'.

| The science of Ayurveda

Ayurveda is an ancient science, which was and still is used to maintain health and wellbeing throughout Indian civilization. Especially in rural areas where there is little money and allopathic (mainstream pharmaceutical) medicine isn't readily available, Ayurveda is used to heal.

Like all indigenous cultures, the wise men and healers had knowledge of the natural world and its ability to cure disease. Their greatest teacher was nature and the five elements: earth, water, fire, air and space. **In Ayurveda, knowledge of the nature of the elements is the primary tool used to work with disease.**

Every human being has all five elements within them, but rather than being distributed equally, they combine in different ways and amounts to make up our individual constitution called our dosha; this includes genetic factors as well as environmental and societal.

To understand each element a little better, let's explore their qualities:

Space is open, endless, empty, light and subtle.

Air is light, moving, changing, dry, rough and also subtle.

Fire is hot, penetrating, transformative, liquefying and intense.

Water is smooth, heavy, lubricating, cohesive and mutable.

Earth is stable, dense, structured, slow and heavy.

Each element doesn't live in isolation. It works with the other elements both to create the body and enable it to function perfectly.

Earth forms our tissues, muscles, bones and the structures of our body.

Water circulates throughout our body in the glandular and circulatory system.

Fire is responsible for all the heat functions in the body like digestion, metabolism and assimilation.

Air has to do with respiration and breathing, and nervous system activity.

Space affects us on a microscopic level as the space in our cells.

Each element likes to gravitate towards its neighbouring element. Kind of like playmates in the school yard who enjoy each other's company because they have interests in common.

Space and **Air** are both light, subtle, intangible elements and form **Vata dosha.**

Fire is all heat and shares the liquefying and spreading qualities of **Water** to form **Pitta dosha.**

Water and **Earth** share a slow, dense, heavy quality, which forms **Kapha dosha.**

Each element likes to gravitate towards its neighbouring element. Kind of like playmates in the school yard who enjoy each other's company because they have interests in common.

The three doshas **Vata**, **Pitta** and **Kapha** combine in our bodies in varying amounts. That's what makes our physiology so unique. We can't be exactly one third Vata, one third Pitta or one third Kapha because our DNA is unique. Usually two doshas predominate with a lesser amount of the third. It's rarer to have just one dosha predominate or to have all three in near equal amounts.

And to mix it up a bit more. Your mind can predominate in one dosha, while your physical body is another dosha. For example, you might have an incredibly quick mind (Vata) while your body frame is a little heavier due to bigger and heavier bones (Kapha).

Constitution is then divided further.

You have the constitution you were born with, like the indelible whorl of your fingerprint. Then you have a current condition; what's presenting right now based on health, lifestyle, emotions, environment, upbringing and so on. In Sanskrit, your birth constitution is called your prakruti and your current condition is called your vikruti.

So how does your prakruti morph into your vikruti?

This is where it gets interesting.

I'll use myself as an example. My birth constitution is Pitta (the fire element) with less Vata and even less Kapha. As a child, teenager and young adult, I was fiery and passionate, determined and liked to be the leader amongst my friends. Physically, I would tend to get overheated and had rashes, fevers, strep throats, while my digestion tended towards loose stools. I had temper tantrums and was easily angered.

When I was pregnant in my twenties and in the early years of bringing up my son, my body became softer and rounder. I put on weight and led a more sedentary existence. I learned to slow down and be patient. I spent more time at home focusing on cooking for my family. This increased the Kapha (the water and earth element) in my system.

In my thirties, when we moved to New York City and I started working full-time teaching yoga from 6 a.m. till 9 p.m., working on weekends and grabbing food on the go, my condition changed again and I suffered from anxiety, constipation, bloating, feeling spacey and had chronic insomnia; all symptoms of an excess of the air and space elements characterised in Vata dosha.

Whenever we are looking at the disease state, we are diagnosing the current condition, the vikruti. In Ayurveda, balance returns when we bring the current condition back to the birth constitution; the vikruti back to the prakruti.

From an Ayurvedic point of view, type 1 and type 2 diabetes are not seen to be related to a particular constitution, i.e. type 1 being Vata/Pitta and type 2 being Kapha. Instead, the constitution is diagnosed first and then treatment varies accordingly.

For example, your constitution could be Pitta/Vata and you could have type 1 diabetes. However, you might show up as more Kapha-dominant because you take insulin, which in turn can tend to store extra fat. When the Kapha is brought back into balance, you may lose weight, have more energy and need less insulin.

Right now, these words Vata, Pitta and Kapha probably don't mean that much to you. So let's explore the doshas and their physical, mental and emotional characteristics a little more deeply to get a feel for which type you might be.

Usually, a questionnaire is used as well as pulse diagnosis by an Ayurvedic practitioner to determine your constitution. Why? Because when we hear the descriptions of our character, we get biased and choose what we'd like to be rather than what we actually are! I've included a basic questionnaire so you can get a rough idea of your vikruti regardless of what type of diabetes you have. If you're curious, go ahead and take the test before you read the descriptions of each dosha coming up next.

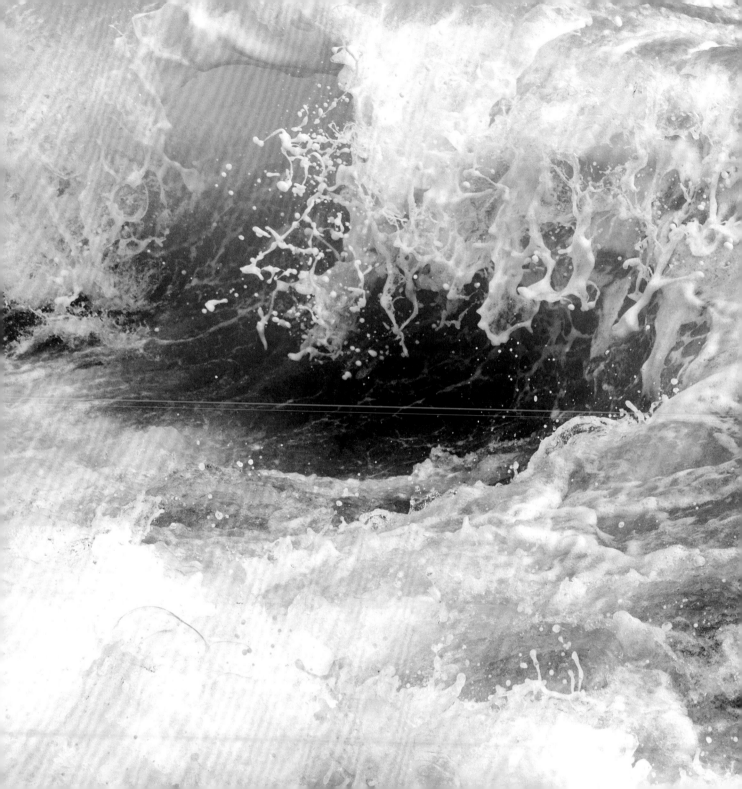

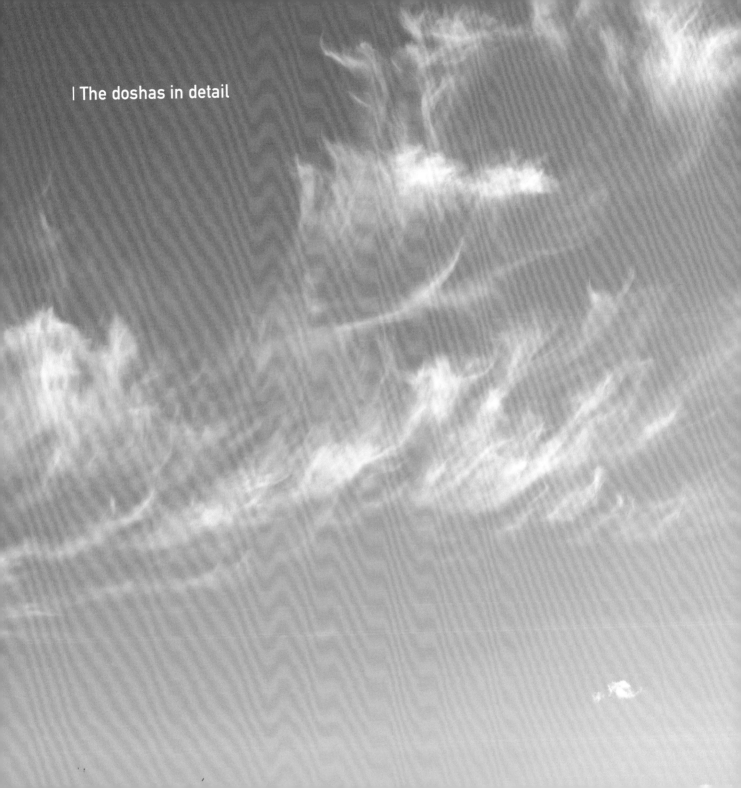

The doshas in detail

VATA DOSHA

Are you always on the go?
Enthusiastic, light-hearted and
sensitive? Do you find yourself
getting ungrounded, overwhelmed
and easily stressed for no reason?
Are you naturally tall and thin or
small and slim?

When I think of **Vata**, what comes to mind is an 'ideas person.' They never stop having ideas and their enthusiasm is contagious. They're the perpetual free spirit and can't stand to be tied to anything. They are constantly on the move and at their best are highly inspirational. We all know them; artists, writers, poets, dancers, musicians and visionaries, who all seem to capture inspiration out of nowhere. We admire them, want to be like them.

But if we are one? That's another story!

The upside is they're never bored. The downside? They get flighty, have trouble following through on their ideas and suffer from fear of failure. When Vata predominates, life is either an incredible ride or a frightening rollercoaster.

Physically, their bodies are light and thin. Veins and bones are easily seen through the skin and teeth can be uneven and sharp. Metabolism is fast and they can have trouble gaining weight. Eyes may dart rapidly in conversation and often the muscles twitch involuntarily. The seat of Vata is in the colon and the predominating element is air which means Vatas suffer from constipation and gas.

Mentally, they are super-sharp and tend towards an overactive mind. They suffer from anxiety and insomnia. Always being on the go means they don't know how to slow down. They rush their meals, forget to eat and ignore signs to slow down and nurture themselves.

If you're starting to feel that I'm talking about you, you might be right. And you might not even be a Vata-dominant constitution.

Today, just about everybody has a Vata imbalance because of our fast-paced society, the demands of technology and our toxic environment.

No one is sleeping enough, eating well or able to enjoy life like they'd like too. The life we want seems out of reach. Put an incurable disease in the mix? We're finished!

So why is everyone Vata imbalanced when we have the other doshas in our constitution as well? Why aren't we all Kapha imbalanced or Pitta imbalanced?

One of the vital systems that relates to the Vata constitution is the nervous system. Keeping the nervous system balanced is a key ingredient in managing stress.

Think about air and space and their qualities. Air and space are intangible. We can't feel space but we can feel air. When the wind hits, our skin dries out and feels rough. But what happens when wind meets wind? It creates more wind, a tornado, a cyclone. When wind meets fire? A forest fire burning out of control. When wind meets water? Huge waves at sea. And finally when wind meets earth? A dust storm. Whatever element wind meets increases the nature of that element. In Ayurveda, Vata is seen as the first dosha to go out of balance and it's the Vata we want to calm and soothe for the good of all the other doshas. No matter what your condition or disease, it's good to nourish and replenish yourself.

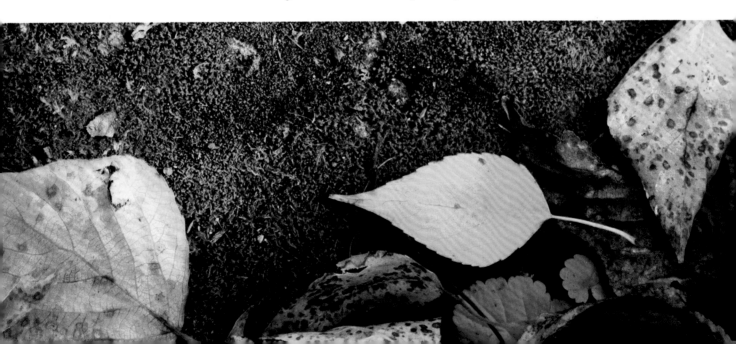

| The key words for Vata

RHYTHM
NOURISHING
CALMING
GROUNDING

Think of the Vata constitution as a butterfly: light, free, delicate, sensitive and incredibly beautiful. In balance, it thrives on the movement of the winds. Out of balance, it can't land and ground, loses focus, and can't find home.

One of the vital systems that relates to the Vata constitution is the nervous system. Keeping the nervous system balanced is a key ingredient in managing stress. If Vata predominates in your constitution, you'll need to be extra careful when it comes to managing your health. Unlike the other doshas, you are less sturdy. That's not always a bad thing. There are many pros to being Vata: you never stay in a bad mood for long; you're quick to go out of balance but quick to come back into balance; your increased sensitivity makes you more intuitive; you recognize when you're unbalanced, and can easily make the effort to rebalance and ground. Most importantly, you thrive when you are loved and nurtured by yourself and others. Love and care go a long way to supporting you in feeling safe and secure.

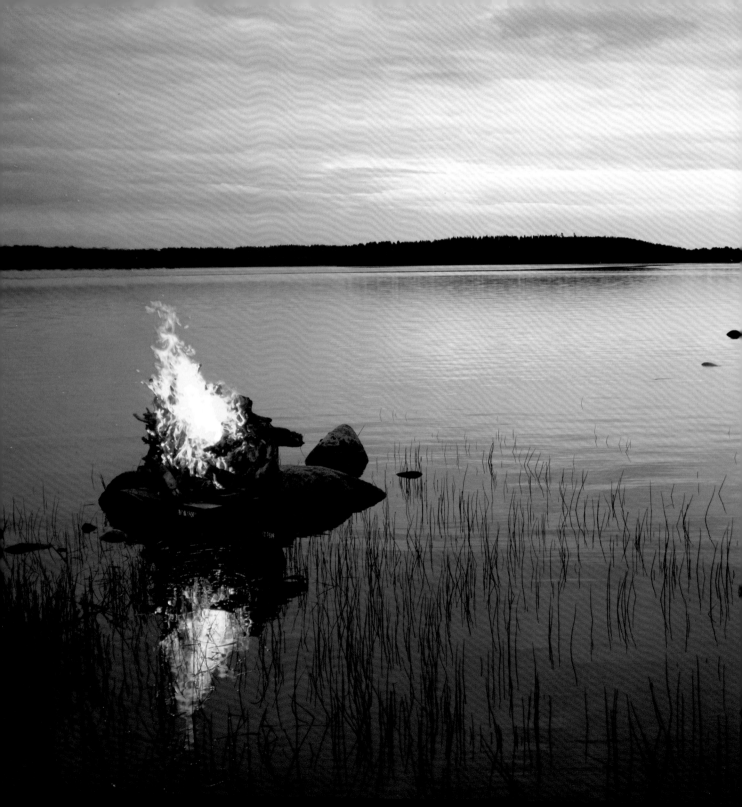

PITTA DOSHA

Are you focused, organized and detail-orientated? Do you find yourself getting overheated and frustrated or burnt out when working hard? Are you strong and sturdy with well-distributed muscle?

Whenever I think of **Pitta**, I think of 'the boss.' It's someone who knows exactly how they like things done. They're good at taking the visionary energy of Vata and directing it into a solid plan. In fact, they are masters of routine and order and are highly capable. A Pitta personality is comfortable in a leadership role, and charismatic, radiant and admired by their peers. At their best, they thrive on completing intricate and challenging tasks; they love a physical challenge and have the constitution of an ox.

At their worst, they are pig-headed, arrogant, competitive, egotistical and take on way more than they should. They don't know how to delegate because they like to hold onto tight control, which often leads to burnout and overwhelm. Usually seen as over-achievers, they think they can take on the world, but then they often come crashing down. Rather than suffering from depression, they feel frustrated and restless.

Pittas thrive when they're occupied whether that's physically through daily exercise or mentally through planning and organizing.

Their physique is usually strong, well-built with good musculature. They're the people we see at the gym, our runners and athletes. It's because of their strong constitution and physical strength that they push themselves to the limit. The seat of Pitta rests in the digestive organs like the stomach, gallbladder, liver and small intestine. This provides them with a good appetite and hardy digestion. They need to eat regularly or they become irritable. Their hair is often red and may be curly. They tend to go bald or grey early. The skin is dappled with moles and freckles and sensitive to the sun. But they love hot environments like saunas, steam rooms, hot baths and sun-bathing!

Mentally, they like everything to be ordered. They abhor chaos. They're the ones with the sweaters and suits neatly arranged in the closet. They take notes with color-coded pencils and are either meticulously on time for appointments or arrive early to ensure they couldn't possibly be late. Pittas find it hard to stand in another person's shoes and expect the same diligence from everyone else. It bugs them when someone else is sloppy, lazy, late or ungrounded. They are the least tolerant of the doshas. They have tons of fire, which serves as their drive and passion. But it literally sears those who don't see things their way.

| The key words for Pitta

FLOWING
COOLING
SOOTHING
DISPERSING

Pittas need to learn how to delegate, ask for support and rest in between intense periods of activity and projects. Rather than eating chillies, garlic, onions (anything deemed as a spicy food) and running in the hot sun at midday, they'd benefit from a cool forest walk at sunset or a swim. Cultivating their playful side is a must as they can get overly serious with just about anything. Pittas thrive when they can explore the qualities of surrender, devotion, service and humility.

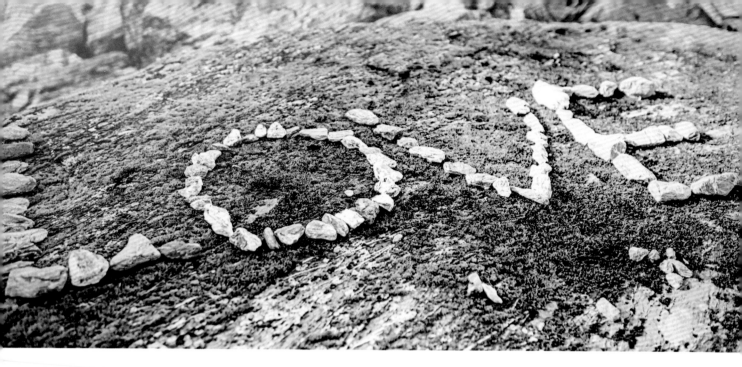

Create beauty in nature, feel love and be loving, allow yourself to feel deeply..

If you're breaking a sweat while reading this or feeling a little hot under the collar, you definitely have some Pitta in you. When Pitta goes out of balance, the body responds by breaking out in a rash, stools loosen and the digestion becomes acidic causing constant burning, burping or ulcers. Pittas' main concern is high blood pressure, heart attack and stroke, the kind of issues that happen suddenly through overexertion, stress and trying too hard.

But don't panic! Being Pitta means you're extremely practical, into longevity and like to have your health under wraps. If anything, you get stressed when it seems like you can't manage your lifestyle.

When a Pitta visits the healthcare provider, they've already collated their symptoms and diagnosed themselves. That's why the practitioner usually has to take the upper hand and show them who's who. If they didn't, they might not be able to emphasize the importance of taking a step back, breathing and letting someone else take out the trash every now and then.

KAPHA DOSHA

Are you someone who feels great after a physical exercise but finds it hard to have the motivation to go in the first place? Do you have bigger bones and tend to notice your digestion is slow? Do you approach your work in a methodical matter, having more patience and tolerance than your friends and workmates?

Kaphas are the ideal friend. They are loyal, trustworthy, compassionate and wonderful at taking a task and following it through to completion. A Vata can throw a million ideas out there, a Pitta will catch and direct them, while the Kapha type has the patience and diligence to bring the projects to fruition.

Kaphas are grounded, have strong, resilient constitutions and aren't easily stressed out. Kaphas have bigger bodies and bone structure, glowing skin, thick hair and lustrous doe-like eyes. Their larger frame affords slightly more padding, and although it's unhealthy for a Kapha to diet, they need to watch their weight. The seat of Kapha is in the chest and the upper third of the stomach. Their energy tends to stagnate there and they may suffer from asthma and breathing problems as well as poor circulation. Their joints are often hyper-mobile and the musculature is often large and soft.

Emotionally, Kaphas are incredibly loving. They forgive easily and like having fun. They have a loving touch and make great caregivers. Mentally, they can sometimes be slow learners, but that's not a bad thing; it means they take great care in understanding a subject before communicating or sharing it with others. They don't have compulsive behavior but they can take things a little too easy. They tend towards overindulgence. Too much wine, women and song! Their big nemesis is laziness, which leads to lethargy and depression. They tend to be possessive and hang onto people and things. The Kaphas are our hoarders with closets stuffed full of mementos and keepsakes.

| The key words for Kapha

HEATING
MOVING
ENERGIZING
RELEASING

Kaphas love to sit and be. It's easy for them to be still and do nothing. But they come alive when there is stimulation, movement and change in their lives. They thrive on exercise. It brings lightness, builds muscle and ignites an inner fire to clear out stagnant energy. Because they like to hang onto things, movement and change are essential. Rather than be a stickler for routine, they need to change it up, shake it up and go wild! Their eating habits can be the biggest challenge as they are attracted to rich foods. They benefit from eating smaller, lighter meals, vigorous daily exercise and lots of mental stimulation.

When a Kapha steps into the Ayurvedic clinic, the doctor will inspire them to take up a diversity of activities, from a spring cleanse and modified diet, to an exercise routine that includes strong breathing practices. As they love people, having a companion to cycle or go to the gym with is a great way to get them up and running. The more you give a Kapha to do, the more they can do and the better they feel.

Express yourself physically get outside, enjoy the sun and light of life..

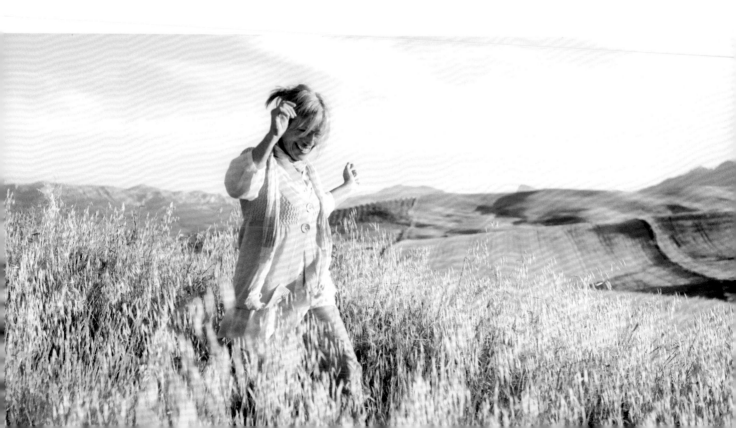

| Putting it all together

After hearing a little about each dosha, you may feel you're all of them. That's because the doshas don't exist in isolation. However, the varying amounts and mix of elements do determine your current condition. When we're at our optimum and feel great, it shouldn't matter what the current condition is. It's when we are imbalanced that it's useful to know what your tendencies are.

One of the key principles of Ayurveda is that the opposite quality brings you back into balance. Think of it like this: if you're feeling cold, you wouldn't take off all your clothes and eat ice cream; you'd put on a sweater, have a hot shower and eat soup.

I can't keep track of how many times I have let my stress get the better of me. Already feeling tired and overwhelmed, I'll stay up late and do that extra task, thinking if I get it over and done with now I'll have more time tomorrow. But tomorrow never comes. Waking up exhausted, my to-do list has grown overnight. When I should be saying no, I feel under pressure to say yes!

Each dosha thrives when the opposing qualities are introduced:

Vata being composed of **Air and Space** needs **Water, Earth and Fire**.
Pitta being composed of **Fire** (and a small amount of **Water**) needs **Water and Earth**.
Kapha being composed of **Earth and Water** needs **Fire, Air and Space**.

Looking at this from a health perspective:

Vata feels calm and nurtured when warm, stable and supported.
Pitta feels soothed when rested, cool and flowing.
Kapha feels alive when motivated, light and stimulated.

Finally, let's explore how the doshas combine uniquely in each person, remembering certain aspects like our physical characteristics (such as bone structure, eye shape, diameter of chest) don't change that much over time and are rarely affected by external factors, whereas emotional, mental characteristics can and do change radically in one lifetime.

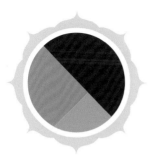

In the pie chart above, the constitution is Pitta/Vata (Kapha). Pitta is dominant both physically, mentally and emotionally, then Vata comes next, with Kapha having least influence.

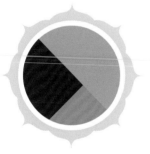

In this pie, however, it's Kapha that is dominant, with less Pitta and hardly any Vata.

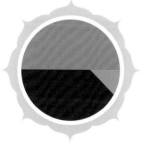

In this pie, we can see that there's equal Pitta and Vata, but with only a tiny bit of Kapha.

To determine your constitution (prakruti), we observe what has remained constant over time, including set personality traits. The questionnaire involves a scoring system where physical traits are given a number of points in each category and the same for mental/emotional traits. The final score determines what percentage you have of each dosha. My first Ayurvedic teacher described it like seeing sections of an apple pie divided up in unequal portions.

These charts illustrate some of the possible constitutional combinations. The combinations are endless but the seven basic ones are written in the following abbreviations.

V/P (k) K/P (v) V/P/K P/V (k) K/V (p) P/K (v) V/K (p)

When the doshas are nearly even, your constitution would be called tridoshic (Vata/Pitta/Kapha). Usually someone who is tridoshic is less likely to have one dosha go easily out of balance. However, if you're pushing the envelope, something's gonna give. Once one of your doshas goes out of balance, it's much harder to bring it back into balance. For example, if you're Vata imbalanced, then balancing it with Pitta and Kapha herbs, diet or lifestyle changes could further imbalance the Pitta and Kapha in your system as well. If you are tridoshic, the ideal prevention and treatment would be to live moderately.

The accompanying questionnaire (p.156) is designed to support you in discovering your current condition as that's what we are dealing with when affected by disease. You'll use the results to design a practice that's perfect for you. You might come back to the questionnaire over time as your health changes. Shifts in time, season, medication, diet or environment will affect you too and determine how the practice can be altered depending on your condition. Your body is a changing system and your practice needs to shift accordingly.

Why not answer the questions now and get your results before reading the next section?

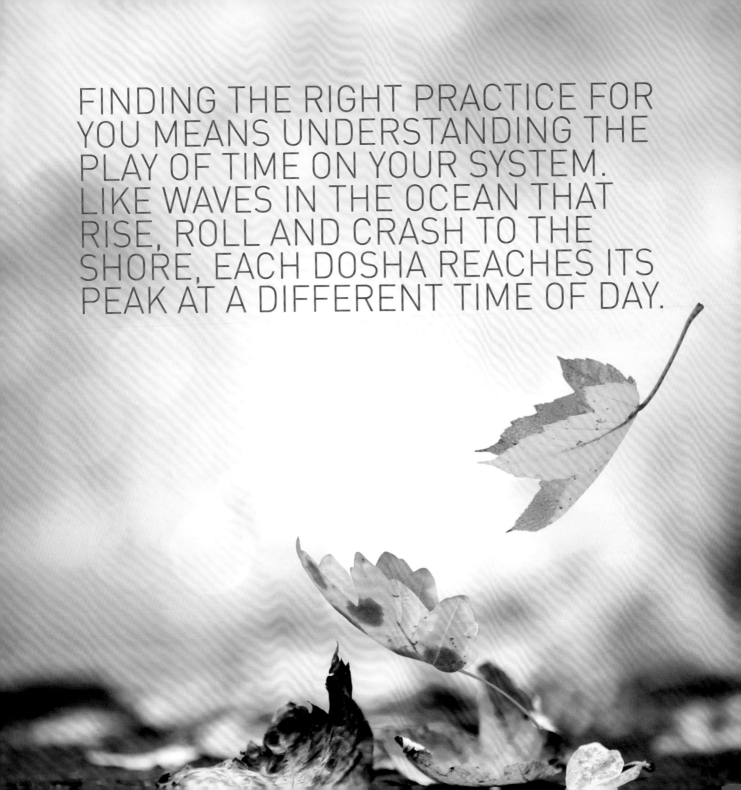

FINDING THE RIGHT PRACTICE FOR YOU MEANS UNDERSTANDING THE PLAY OF TIME ON YOUR SYSTEM. LIKE WAVES IN THE OCEAN THAT RISE, ROLL AND CRASH TO THE SHORE, EACH DOSHA REACHES ITS PEAK AT A DIFFERENT TIME OF DAY.

| A season for everything

Have you ever noticed how there seems to be a vibe to different parts of the day? Or how your body and mind react to the different seasons? Even the stage of life that you're in determines how you respond mentally, physically and emotionally to the external world.

As you explore the practice that's right for you in managing your diabetes, it's useful to understand each dosha and its relationship to the seasons, the time of day, and stage of life.

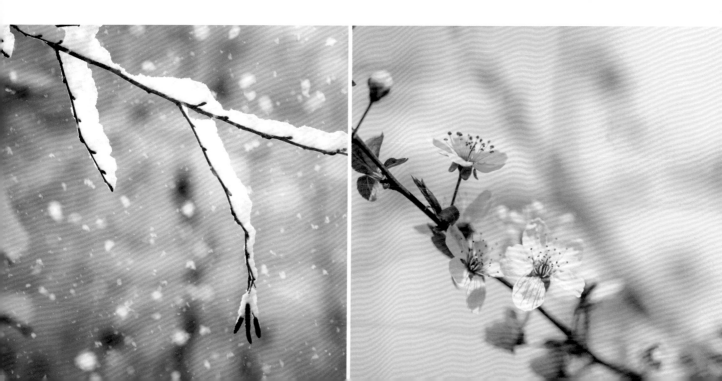

Vata season

Vata builds during late summer, then overflows through autumn, generally from equinox, then peaks as it comes to winter solstice. It's also the point when a lot of people get colds and flu. One minute the weather is warming up; the next it's freezing cold and snowing again.

During Vata season, you can struggle more with maintaining good blood glucose (BG) levels. Just when everything seems balanced, you catch a cold or get that unexpected sunburn. The rapid changes become stressors rather than motivators. This is a great time go to bed a little earlier, enjoy staring into the light of a fire, dream and let yourself be lulled by the warmth of family and friends. During Vata season, it's also beneficial to start a regular yoga practice that includes grounding postures as well as relaxing forward bends and restorative poses. Regardless of your dominant dosha, be more vigilant about your health during autumn and winter.

Here are 4 simple ways you can minimize stress in Vata season:

1. Dress in layers, carry an umbrella and scarf, and be prepared for changes in the weather.

2. Make sure your skin is moisturized, especially your feet.

3. Eat warm, nurturing foods with warming spices like ginger, cinnamon, cardamom, turmeric, fennel, even a bit of cooked onion to bring in the sweet element.

4. Keep a regular routine. Get up at the same time every day and go to bed at the same time at night. Having a regular meal routine (eating at the same times each day) will help the body know when to fire up the digestion.

Kapha season

Kapha builds during winter, then overflows/aggravates during the spring, especially as the first rains come. The colder and drier weather, which eventually turns to the unpredictability of spring, means we need to not only stay warm but be prepared for sudden changes, such as cold one minute, wet and warm the next.

Colder weather affects circulation and can have an effect on BG levels. If you feel sluggish, it's the perfect time to start an exercise regime. Head to the gym, go for walks and grab the sunshine when you can. Avoid heavy, stale and processed foods as they tend to stagnate the energy in your system. A yoga practice in winter and early spring is stimulating, with more backbends and heating inversions as well as balancing and standing postures to develop strength and stamina.

There are 3 simple guidelines to get the best from Kapha season:

1. Get outside, exercise and organize activities with friends.

2. Eat warm nourishing foods that don't weigh you down.

3. Keep your skin nourished and add stimulating scents like rosemary, pine and sage.

Pitta season

Summer! It's hot and sultry and you stay up late. In Pitta season, passion and tension runs hot. Summer means holidays, time in the sun and water.

Our BG levels fluctuate because of less sleep and more social outdoor activities. The hot weather can be aggravating as much as it's pleasurable. Cooling activities and foods are recommended. Avoid overstimulation. Find ways to soothe and nurture your system. Avoid doing anything in the midday sun. It's a great time for salads, but make sure to include oily dressings or an avocado. Take a cool shower as opposed to a hot bath. Keep your skin hydrated with nourishing coconut oil. Pitta season is a great time to put down your to-do list and play. Enjoy the little things. Don't sweat the big things. A yoga practice includes lots of forward bends, restorative poses and rest between the more active postures.

Follow these 4 simple steps to get the most out of Pitta season:

1. Keep cool and calm.

2. Make everything you do fun - being playful is more important than being right!

3. Avoid heating activities, too much sun, hot baths and steam rooms.

4. Eat cooling foods and stay hydrated!

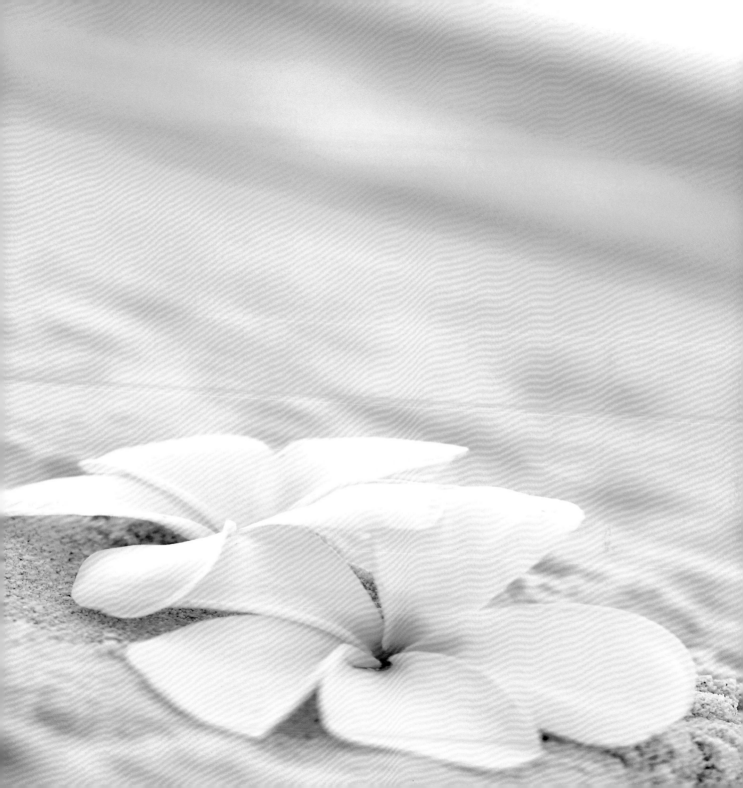

| The perfect time of day

Like the seasons, the time of day is divided into Vata, Pitta and Kapha. According to research into exercise physiology, blood sugar levels increase and decrease at different times of the day. So far, I haven't found any anecdotal studies on how time of day, blood sugar levels and the doshas relate, but it may be interesting for you to observe your own levels and notice the influence that the time of day and its doshic equivalent has on your BG levels.

Pre-dawn

2 a.m. to 6 a.m. is when Vata predominates. If you tend to wake up at 2 a.m. or 3 a.m., there might be too much Vata in the system. This kind of insomnia is no fun as it can bring on anxiety and restlessness. Dreams can be disturbing and filled with irrational fears and unlikely scenarios. In Ayurveda, waking before 6 a.m. is ideal. Prana (the Sanskrit term for life force energy) is still low to the earth and easily absorbed. A simple breathing practice performed pre-dawn is nourishing for the nervous system.

Morning routines

6 a.m. until 10 a.m. is when Kapha predominates. It's the perfect time for morning routines and exercise. You can utilize the energies of the earth and water elements by performing grounding physical activities and implementing simple Ayurvedic cleansing practices that stimulate and invigorate your body. Breakfast should be simple and light, so the mind is fresh for the workday ahead.

Lunch time

10 a.m. to 2 p.m. is when Pitta predominates. Your digestive fire is at its highest. It's the best time to eat your biggest meal of the day, which could be a late breakfast, brunch or lunch. During the heat of the day avoid heavy exercise, sun and stressful work-related activities. This gives your body the chance to digest its food.

Afternoon rest

2 p.m. to 6 p.m. is Vata time again. Ever feel like you struggle to stay awake in the afternoons? Have difficulty concentrating? Is your child grumpy? Does your baby cry? In the afternoons, Vata peaks and creates a sense of either restlessness, hyperactivity or total exhaustion. Why not take a nap and/or do something creatively stimulating? Remember how Vata thrives on ideas? Letting go of the restless feelings by taking time out can bring on the next surge of creative inspiration.

Bed time

6 p.m. to 10 p.m. Kapha returns. In the evening, Kapha's slower more nurturing quality promotes a sense of peace and relaxation. Take your time to cook food. Go for a walk after dinner. Practice yoga, listen to music, watch a favorite movie and get to bed before 10 p.m. Falling asleep in Kapha time means your rest will be deep and restorative.

The midnight hour

10 p.m. until 2 a.m. is when Pitta rises while we sleep. It digests all the thoughts and ideas from the day. It heals the body enabling us to push the reset button. If you eat after 10 p.m., you're diverting the metabolic system away from its intended function. And when you stay up past 10 p.m., the body longing for sleep is starved of its natural rhythm and produces the stress response hormones cortisol and adrenaline. This overheats and dries the system, damaging all cells, but most particularly the nervous system. You might not notice it at first but getting a good night's sleep is the first step in the management of any disease.

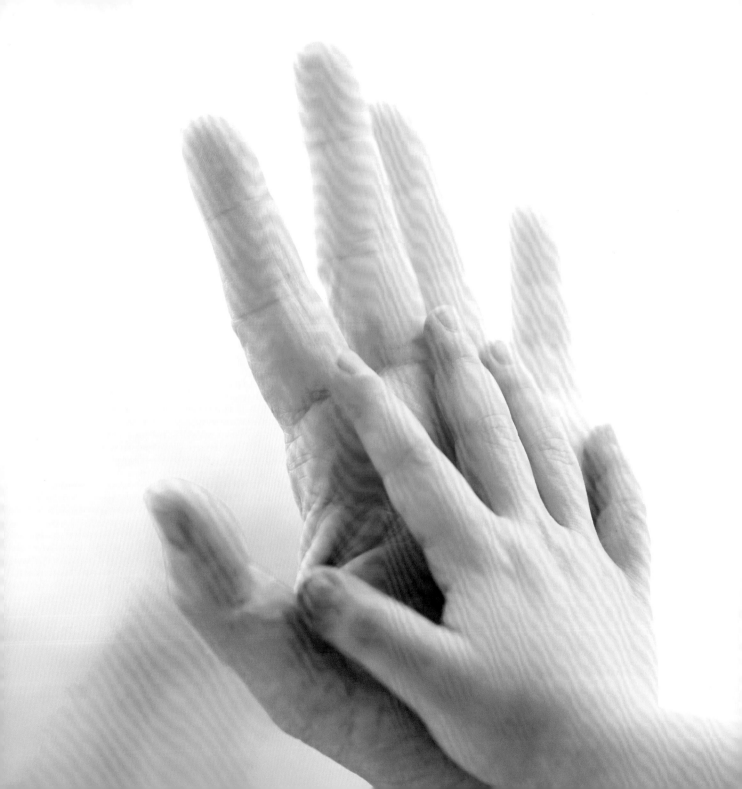

I The stages of life

Each stage of your life has certain characteristics and degrees of awareness. How you felt as a child and how you perceive the world in your teenage years, adulthood and finally old age is completely different. The doshas are divided into three life periods. How you manage the disease over that period will vary according to your dosha and type of diabetes.

Birth to puberty

This stage of life is Kapha. As a baby and young child, you have good immunity. You are unaffected by stress, innocent and naturally loving. Physically active and inquisitive, you thrive on stimulation and adventure. Wearing your heart on your sleeve, you express emotions freely.

As hard as it is to see a child affected by disease, their response and coping mechanism is often remarkable. They manage much better than an adult does. They haven't fully identified with the illness because the ego isn't developed enough to take ownership of the disease. They are fearless and brave.

Puberty through to menopause or retirement

This stage of life is Pitta. In adulthood, your inner fire kicks in. You strive towards success and enjoy hard work and physicality. You want to achieve goals in life and look for a partner, a home and a successful career. The Pitta years are full of activity and diversity.

The heat of a growing life gives rise to stress and difficulties. It's much harder for us to slow down because life is pushing us forward. Like the Pitta personality type, this stage of life is relentless. Society places its pressures on us and we feel we must be successful or else! No wonder we find ourselves burnt out, stressed and unwell. As adults, we struggle to understand the importance of rest and play, key ingredients from our childhood.

The elder years

This stage of life is Vata. Once children have grown and work responsibilities have diminished, you begin to focus on meaningful pursuits. Life literally feels lighter! Time to take up a creative hobby, travel more, do what you didn't have time for during your 20s, 30s, 40s and even 50s.

In our elder years, we must be more attentive to the changes happening physically, mentally and emotionally. The physical structures of the body like our bones and tissues become drier, eyesight and hearing diminishes, memory is no longer acute. We sleep less and are prone to Vata imbalances like insomnia and anxiety. Slowing down, taking our time, rhythm, routine, doing what we love and making meaningful health and lifestyle choices go a long way in enabling us to feel vibrant and fulfilled in our later years.*

As the picture unfolds of your unique type, the rhythm of the days, seasons and ages, it's easy to understand why a disease like diabetes is so complex and unpredictable. Your approach, attitude, medications and diet will constantly change from when you have diabetes as a child and your parents supported you in daily management to when you become a teenager, adult, then elderly person. Knowing what to add when can be confusing. Not to mention the how. Put fear of complications into the mix, plus emotions and a host of environmental and societal pressures? It's a wonder we aren't all basket cases.

Miraculously, we aren't. In fact, having a disease that demands a regime, something Pitta types thrive on and Vata and Kaphas need, makes us stronger, more capable, accepting and patient. Obviously, it isn't all roses; anger, depression as well as sadness, grief, frustration and burnout are pretty high up there as emotional side effects.

I'd like to suggest that any emotions we encounter when faced with our health arise because we see the disease as standing in the way of our perceived happiness. We all have different definitions of happiness. Think about it for a moment. What's yours? What do you feel stands in the way of your happiness? And how many times do you notice different emotions coming up when you don't get what you want?

A deep understanding of yourself as an individual, your natural reactions and concerns is relevant in taking the first steps to feeling better about your diagnosis.

Because diabetes is such an unpredictable disease, it's hard to trust in a definitive outcome. This creates instability in the mind. The mind is wonderful at taking in information and labelling it. Every experience is neatly filed away and can be relived at any time. The part of the mind that defines and categorizes is different to the part of the mind that takes in information. One is intellect and the other is merely a feedback mechanism. What happens when the intellect can't make sense of the information? We get confused! It's like trying to put what's entering your world into a box, only to find that the box is missing. And what happens when we can't resolve a thought, experience or situation? Depression, anxiety and associated emotional and mental disorders rear their ugly heads.

A deep understanding of yourself as an individual, your natural reactions and concerns is relevant in taking the first steps to feeling better about your diagnosis. The science of Ayurveda enables you to see things more objectively, gives you a language to navigate your moods and supports you to work with a practice that's just right for whatever comes up.

*If you want to explore this subject further I highly recommend you visit an Ayurvedic practitioner or pick up one of the books on the recommended reading list in the resources section at the back of the book.

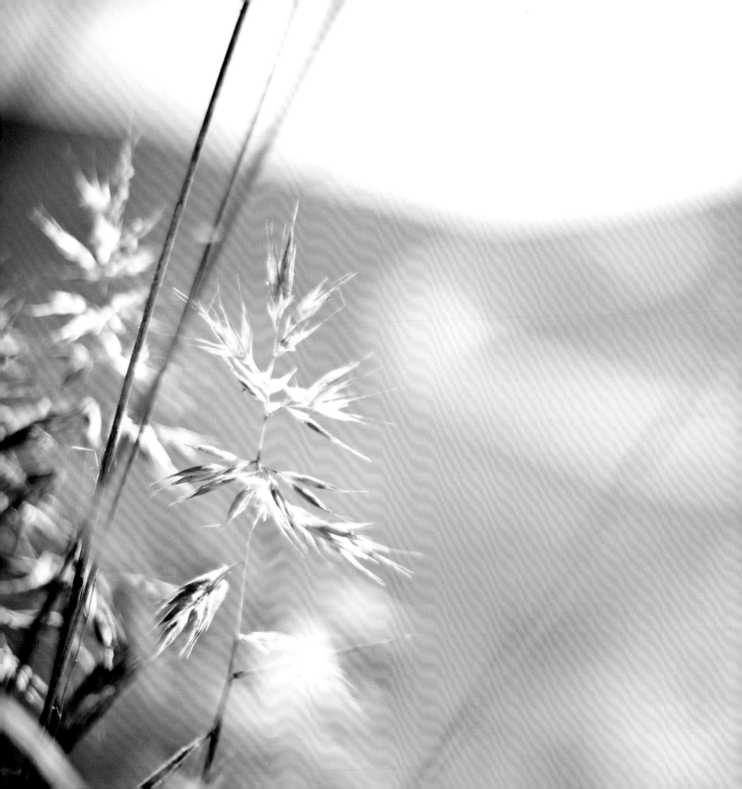

Now that you know your current condition, understand the best times of day to practice, have observed what season of the year it is and your age, how does that all work with the type of diabetes you have?

In Ayurveda, diabetes is classified into the three doshas. Vata diabetes is divided into 4 types, Pitta diabetes into 6 types, and Kapha diabetes into 10. These different types of diabetes are classified according to the urine, its volume and what's being excreted through the urine. The way we respond to insulin, diet and lifestyle is affected by our current condition. That same current condition determines whether the disease is curable or incurable.

| The doshas and your type of diabetes

That means, besides being a person with Vata, Pitta or Kapha diabetes, you can have:

Kapha/Pitta diabetes
Kapha/Vata diabetes
Pitta/Vata diabetes
Vata/Pitta/Kapha diabetes

In general, the symptoms of diabetes for all doshas and types are: excessive urination, thirst and lethargy. However, each dosha has its own set of unique symptoms, which can be grouped like this.

Kapha symptoms: indigestion, loss of appetite, a tendency to vomit, excessive sleep, cough and frequent colds with a runny nose.

Pitta symptoms: pain in bladder and urethra, pain in testes, fever, burning sensation, thirst, acidity, dizziness, loose stools, pain in the heart area, insomnia.

Vata symptoms: feeling ungrounded, twitches and shaking, gripping sensation in the chest, empathy, pain, insomnia, weight loss, cough, difficulty breathing and constipation.

The disease is further classified as: curable, manageable or incurable.

When the disease is caught early (pre-diabetes, type 2 diabetes), it's categorized as a Kapha disease. The person might be overweight and has lifestyle habits which increase BG levels. It's seen as curable because the person can change their lifestyle habits and their BG levels may return to normal.

In people with Pitta and some Kapha symptoms (progressed type 2), the disease is manageable mainly through herbal treatment, diet and lifestyle adjustments.

The incurable versions of diabetes (type 1 and LADA, juvenile and MODY) are inherited. This could be both Pitta and Vata and possibly some Vata/Kapha types. These are only manageable through insulin therapy.

| The role of immunity in diabetes management

In yoga and Ayurveda, immunity is called ojas. Ojas comes from the densest tissue in the body, reproductive fluid. It's the densest tissue because it carries the seed of life. Without reproductive fluid, there would be no propagation of the species. That some of us are born with less immunity than others or develop immune system problems as we age has to do with the loss of ojas. In Ayurveda, it's believed that everyone is born with eight drops, which reside in the heart. The amount of ojas is highly dependent upon the health of our parents at conception. It's easy to lose ojas, but incredibly hard to build once lost.

In a person with a healthy immune system, stress is one of the main factors in the depletion of ojas. We live on a diet of excess food, sex, media and stimulation. In a person with diabetes, stress isn't the only issue. Urination and sweating also contribute to the loss of ojas.

Ojas gets further imbalanced in two ways:

1. Through obstruction in the blood vessels, the excess sugar makes the environment overly acidic and literally corrodes the arteries.

2. Through degeneration of bodily tissues, if the organs aren't receiving the right balance of energy from glucose, they are also impaired.

Ojas fuels our strength to fight illness. It's like armour. Without it, we aren't protected from invaders. In Ayurveda, the treatment of diabetes includes ways to build and maintain ojas. Getting our BG levels under control is the first step. The channels, or srotas as they're called in Ayurveda, direct energy (prana) and nutrients throughout the entire system. They are seen as both gross, i.e. blood vessels and nerves, and subtle energetic pathways. High BG levels block the srotas.

We've been educated on how to manage our levels from an allopathic perspective with a variety of views on diet, insulin dosage and lifestyle approaches. We are encouraged to manage stress, because as someone living with diabetes, it's impossible to change the stressor. (We can't snap our fingers and no longer have diabetes.)

Ayurveda takes a holistic tack and offers treatment specific to your constitution (prakruti), the type of dosha which dominates in the disease state, your current condition (vikruti), the type of obstruction in the srota, your mental constitution, diet, lifestyle habits and genetic factors.

In general, type 1 is treated with nourishing medications and therapies that will build ojas. This includes oil massage, herbal therapies, yoga, breathing and meditation practices alongside insulin therapy and or allopathic medications.

In general, type 2 diabetes (as a disease of excess) is treated with purification therapies, such as vomiting, herbs to induce expulsion of toxins through the bowels, herbal enemas and exercise. The patient is also given a list of dos and don'ts, a daily regime to stimulate the immune system so it can return to vibrant health.

Rather than purporting to be a miracle cure, Ayurveda and yoga offer the perfect solution to manage the energy system that is the body. Knowledge of your body puts the power back in your hands. If you know which dosha is dominant in your current condition, you can self-treat, just like you do when you have a hypo, or need to bolus before or after a meal.

My endocrinologist shared with me that after I'd brought my diabetes under control, my need to see him or get advice would be minimal. "You're in the driver's seat and you'll know what you need to find the perfect balance."

The practices of yoga and the lifestyle guidelines from Ayurveda build and maintain ojas, bringing not only physical strength but strength of will. Think of your willpower like a muscle. You have to exercise it to develop it. Yoga teaches you to take the mind and focus it in on one thing: you. You expressing yourself in the practice as breath, as movement, as flow. The more you bring yourself to the practice, the stronger your willpower and the more you want to practice. In approaching anything new, it takes courage and faith to take the first step.

If you're like me, it isn't easy. I have and do suffer from diabetes burnout. My approach, being a Pitta type, has always been to use frustration as energetic fuel to fire up my practice. The more frustrated I am, the deeper my daily surrender. If you tend to be someone who loses focus, like a Vata, then use your creative inspiration to develop your will. See your yoga practice as an art. Something you explore like colors on a canvas, each day adding a touch of paint here or there until eventually you've got the moves down. And if you're someone who just doesn't get revved up easily, like the Kapha type, enlist a friend to do some of these exercises with you. It's always better and more fun to do things together.

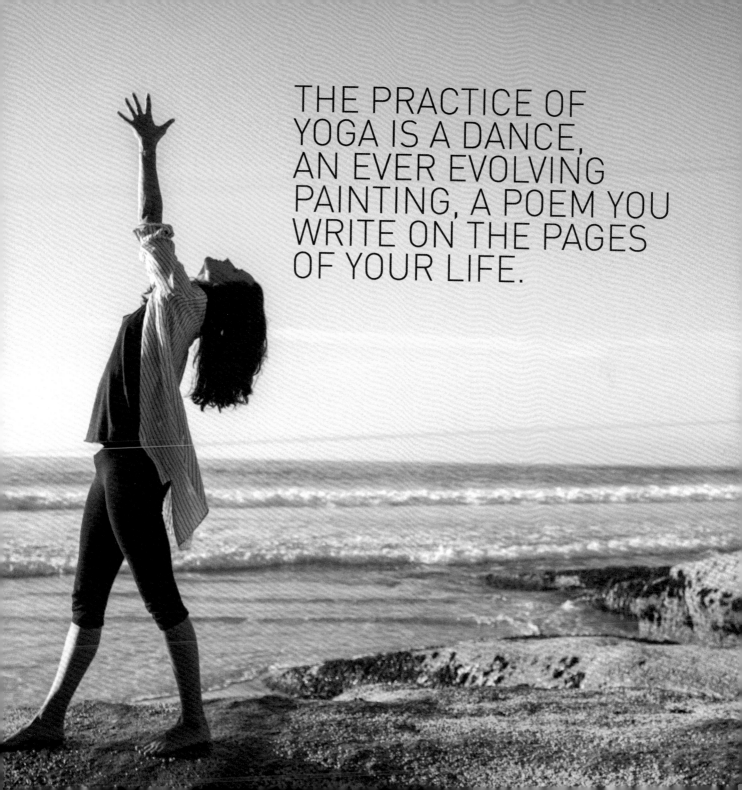

THE PRACTICE OF
YOGA IS A DANCE,
AN EVER EVOLVING
PAINTING, A POEM YOU
WRITE ON THE PAGES
OF YOUR LIFE.

CHAPTER TWO
THE MIND

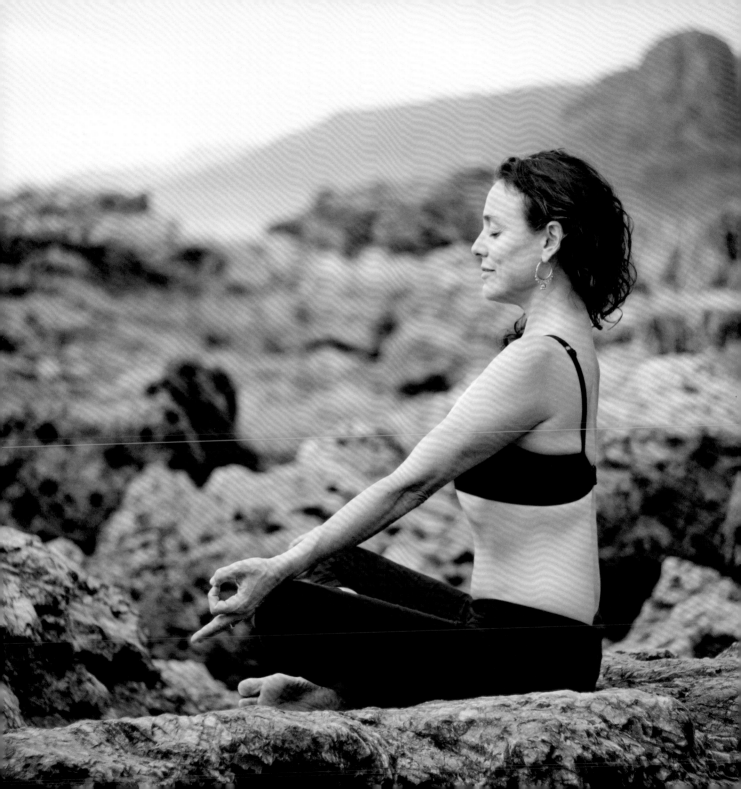

| Thoughts and the mysterious mind

Once you've completed the questionnaire and found out your current condition (or vikruti), you may find yourself fuelled up and inspired to practice. You've most likely fast forwarded to the yoga sequence, breathing and meditation chapter to get an idea of what you're in for. I get it...I'd have done that myself.

But wait!

There's one more factor to consider and understand before diving headlong into starting a daily personalised yoga practice.

Your state of mind.

Your mind is your best friend, the absolute genius in your life. And yet, it's also your worst enemy, when not understood. Armed with a battalion of thoughts that won't let up, we've been conditioned in our lives to see thoughts as 'good' and 'bad'. But here's where I let you in on a little secret.

Thoughts don't work like that.

Thoughts are innocent. They don't have meaning, because they don't exist. Try to catch a thought. To hold onto it. Try to think a thought. How deep, long, wide is a thought? Does it have a shape? How about a size? How long does it last?

These ideas were introduced to me while I was studying the orthodox system of knowledge called Vedanta. And let me tell you, they absolutely revolutionised the way I approach stress.

| So what is a thought?

A thought is a label, a name for a thing you've either seen or experienced, either in present time or filed away in memory.

Everything in your whole life has been named for you. Take a moment. Look around the room. Is there anything that you can see right now that doesn't have a name? Everything in the known universe is known because it's been named. You've even been named! But that doesn't mean you are the name. Were you born with a name? Would you still exist if your name was different? Your parents named you, sure, but for that first year or so of your life, it's likely you didn't even recognize your name. Until eventually it stuck. And then as you got older, you started to look at things and ask your parents the names of those things.

As a baby, not knowing the names of things, no thoughts. Until that first thought comes, which also becomes your first memory. Then eventually your head is full of millions of names, labels, thoughts, which in turn become memories, experiences, ideas and ultimately your belief system.

Thoughts, being names for things, having no dimension of their own, are innocent. They can't be good or bad, positive or negative. You decide to put meaning into a thought. Think of a knife, in the hands of a murderer or in the hands of a surgeon. In one, it's a death sentence; in the other, a lifesaver. It's the person wielding the knife who matters. Every thought is like that. You decide what to do with it. Think of a thought like it's a photograph. Every photograph is placed in an album of memories. Acting on a thought is like opening the album and selecting the photograph.

When we take up a yoga practice and start to bring body, breath and mind together, it's not necessarily going to turn out like what you see on Instagram. In fact, you might feel like you're experiencing the opposite of yoga. A busy mind. Constant distraction. Chatter chatter chatter in your head.

The random arrival of thoughts are like waves in the ocean. They come and go, returning to their source. The source being you!

Relax. Take a breath. It's perfectly normal to feel frustrated and out of your depth. Especially when those pesky thoughts seem to be piling on top of each other to get your attention. As soon as you attempt to focus the mind, every thought that's ever bothered you will rear its ugly head.

A simple example to alleviate your worries is to think of your mind as a device that labels, stores and manages thoughts. Similar to your PC or Mac, each thought, belief, idea and experience is neatly filed yet available at any time. Now, what happens when you stop what you're doing and leave your computer for a few minutes? The screensaver pops up to remind you that the computer is still active. It's the same with your thoughts. When you focus the mind, such as concentrating on one posture or your breath, the mind can no longer identify with a particular thought. So just to remind you that you're still awake, it throws up a random thought.

The random arrival of thoughts are like waves in the ocean. They come and go, returning to their source. The source being you!

It's easy to think that a thought is bugging you, but in reality you're bugging the thought. If you weren't there experiencing the thought, would it matter if the thought was there or not? Of course not. You give life to every thought. And knowing this is key to being able to let go and relax.

On deeper examination, let's take a thought and follow its life span.

Understand that every thought has an address, the address being the final resolution of the thought. You might see something you want, like a piece of chocolate. First the thought comes, "Chocolate." Chocolate on its own is innocent. It's your memory of the experience of chocolate that colors the thought. Then, from that previous experience, desire arises, "I want it." Depending on the level of the desire, you take action. In the action you assume the role of chocolate-getter. And now the thought gains momentum and becomes energy in motion, emotion.

As an emotion the thought becomes dynamic and appears as either good or bad. "I want the chocolate, but I have diabetes" or "My A1c is so good this month, surely I can have a little piece of chocolate". Once the thought is in motion it reaches the address - chocolate - and gets resolved, or it doesn't and stays unresolved. As long as that thought stays unresolved, it hangs around like a ghost in your mind and appears to keep haunting you. And the longer that thought haunts you, the more depressed and frustrated you become.

That's why yoga is the ultimate thought-buster. On a physical level, yoga takes your mind out of its habitual need to identify with thoughts and the need to bring each thought to resolution.

Feeling like you should get rid of or avoid thoughts is not the issue. What's more important? The thought? Or you the thinker? Obviously, it's always going to begin and end with you. And I'm not talking about accepting yourself. You don't need to accept yourself to be aware that you think.

The beautiful thing about being human is that we are conscious of being conscious. We know that we are aware. All of creation is conscious to a greater or lesser degree, but even an animal, who has thoughts, doesn't label its thoughts. Only we humans do that. Animals get lost in thoughts like we do. Have you ever seen a dog with a stick? They spend hours chewing and chasing that thing completely obsessed. Eventually they will drop the stick.

But do we drop a thought?

We make the mistake of thinking that a thought contains the fulfilment of our desires. And around and around we go.

The practices in this book are not a cure-all, nor do they banish thoughts. First, they help us to become aware of thoughts. Next, they support the mind in getting out of its habitual need to identify with thoughts. The peace, harmony and relaxation that you feel after practice is not external to you. It is the nature of who you are.

If you've been to a yoga class, you may have heard the teacher share that yoga is about stopping the thoughts. Or that yoga happens in the space between the breaths. Or that yoga is about being in the moment. These are ideas which create an impossible ideal no matter what your level of experience. I'm here to let you know you can drop all those ideals.

Let your thoughts arise. Don't try to stop them. Follow them if you like. Have fun with your thoughts. See them for what they are and then return to your breath, the posture. Wherever you place your mind, that's where the energy goes.

There's a sweet story in the tradition of Vedanta.

Once there was a boy who met a sage who had a wish-fulfilling monkey. The boy, transfixed by the monkey's powers, begged the Sage for the monkey. The Sage, happy to hand him over, insisted that the boy comply with one condition. The monkey would be his as long as he fed him wishes. If he ran out of wishes, the monkey would devour him. The boy, in his greed, thought nothing of the condition. He was sure he had enough wishes to last three lifetimes. The Sage, not so sure, hid himself in a nearby bush just in case everything took a turn for the worse.

The boy, eager to get the show on the road, made his first wish. Immediately, the object of his desire was there. The boy made another wish. And another. Each time he made a wish, the monkey worked its magic.

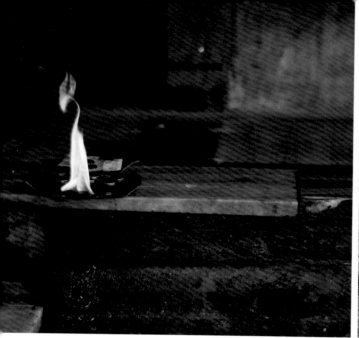

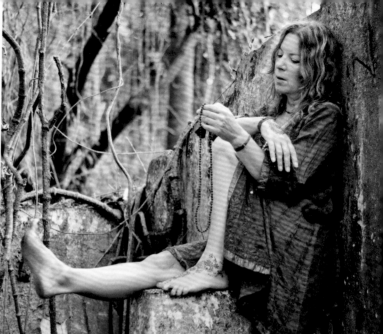

Soon the boy's backyard was littered with cars, boats, trucks, yachts, houses, and more. As soon as he wished, the monkey manifested, until eventually the boy was exhausted and couldn't think of desires fast enough. He began to panic.

As luck would have it, the Sage reappeared and enquired as to how the boy was managing. The boy, relieved to see him, shared that he was exhausted, feared for his life and wondered how the Sage could have ever managed to control the monkey. The Sage smiled and, pointing to a nearby pole, suggested the boy make one last wish.

"You see that pole? Tell the monkey you wish for it to run up and down the pole forever. It will never bother you again."

The story is simple but its meaning profound. When we identify with our thoughts, we bring them to life. But if we give the mind a focus like the breath, a posture or a simple concentration technique, it is happily occupied. When the mind is occupied, there's more energy available for greater health and wellbeing.

CHAPTER THREE
THE BREATH

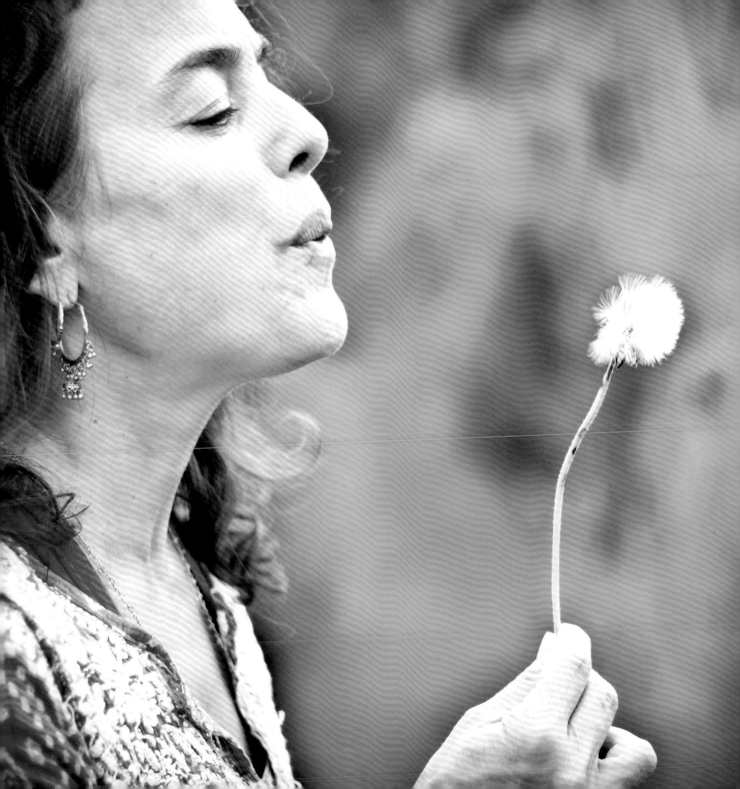

I Taking it one breath at a time

Breath. We can't live without it. So why is it that we forget the most essential ingredient in keeping every single part of the body working properly? I believe it's the very fact that we take breath for granted that's the problem. It's only when we're out of breath that we notice the breath. Like when you have a cold or an allergy and you're gasping for air. That's when you think, "Hang on a second. I'm not breathing all that well."

Instead, if you could take note of what's happening with your breath moment by moment, you'd be surprised. The breath has so many intriguing variations, waves and moods. It's a whole culture unto itself.

I never knew much about the breath until I took up yoga. Whenever we started breathing, I wanted to run a mile. I kept feeling nervous and afraid every time we had to lie back over blankets and breathe. I didn't really trust my body and was convinced that one day I'd get some sort of disease and die. As I mentioned, the impact of my mother's death was huge and unresolved, not only emotionally but physically. It's why I took up yoga in the first place. Yoga was my lifeline, a way to tranquilize all my insecurities and fears, breath being the starting point.

Accessing the breath and learning to breathe fully and deeply became even more of a priority once I found out I had diabetes. When the numbers went up, I took a breath. When the numbers were low, I took a breath. When I felt overwhelmed, I took a breath. When I wanted to cry and scream and disappear... I took a breath.

One of my first teachers stressed that the breath could be manipulated and extended, but only once the body was completely relaxed and aligned. Another teacher said exactly the opposite. insisting that the body and its movements fit around the breath.

Whether the body guides the breath or the breath guides the body, working with the breath is a powerful tool in relaxing the nervous system.

What happens when we breathe?

Before you jump into the asana practice, take the time to understand the mechanics of breathing so that you can confidently bring your breath to every single posture.

Whether the body guides the breath or the breath guides the body, working with the breath is a powerful tool in relaxing the nervous system.

The mechanics of breath are simple. The body expands on inhalation to take in air and the body contracts on exhalation to expel air. You may think it's just your belly or chest that's moving, but when I say 'the body,' I'm talking about a whole dynamic spinal expression that involves muscles, bones and nerves. When the body is full of tension, it's much harder for all these different body parts to work in harmony. Every single part of the mechanism inspires every other part. So holding tension in your chest will force other muscles to do more work. Holding tension in the belly means the chest will have to work harder. And so on.

Physiologically, the most important muscle in breathing is the diaphragm, a sheet of muscle that sits underneath the ribcage in the shape of a dome or upside-down mushroom. The stem of the mushroom is called the central tendon. In a normal breath pattern, when you breathe in, the diaphragm releases down which pushes the belly out. When you breathe out, the diaphragm releases back up again and the belly comes in towards the spine. If the stem of your mushroom is tight, the belly hardly expands and most of the effort for inhalation and exhalation comes from the muscles around the chest. Breathing only in the upper part of the chest indicates stress, but we can calm this through yoga by learning to breathe more fully.

Part of what you want to explore in your yoga practice is how to get the breath full and deep. Many yoga practices emphasise a style of breath called ujjayi breathing. This is a breath that involves constricting the throat and forcing the air to travel through a narrow pathway. It's a cooling breath that develops concentration. However, if you are trying to soothe the nervous system, the full complete breath is ideal.

The different Ayurvedic doshas benefit from different kinds of breath in practice. As you explore the different breathing practices, you'll discover which one suits you best.

| What type of breather are you?

In order to choose the breath that's going to benefit you best, aim to get a sense of what your personal breathing pattern is. Here are some exercises you can try to get more comfortable exploring the breath.

Time: 5 to 10 minutes.

What you'll need:

- A blanket, yoga mat or something comfortable to lie on

- A rolled up towel or blanket for under your head if your chin juts out when you lie on the floor

- Something supportive to place under your knees if you have any lower back issues

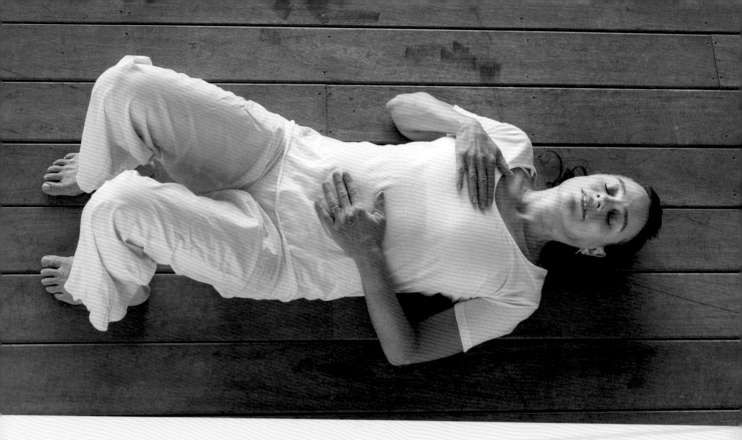

| EXERCISE 1

Lie on the floor on your back with your knees bent and your feet flat on the surface beneath you.

Place one hand on your belly and one on your chest.

Breathe naturally and observe your breath.

Take your time.

Notice: Is it easier to breathe into your chest or your belly?

This breath observation is called natural relaxed breathing.

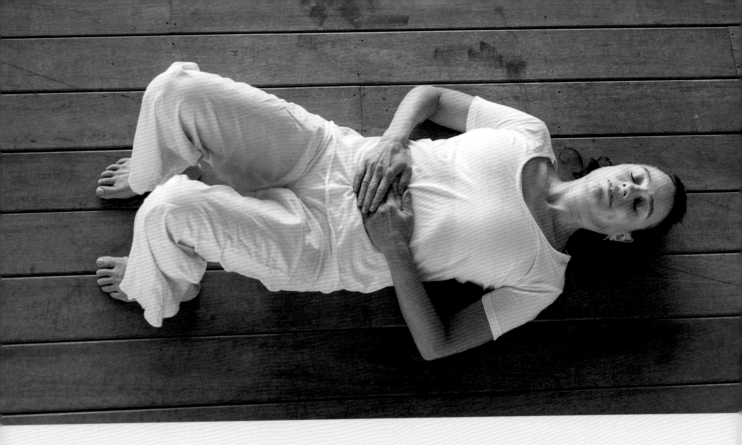

| EXERCISE 2A

Begin with natural relaxed breathing (knees bent, feet flat).
Firmly hold the belly with your hands and try to breathe into
your chest.

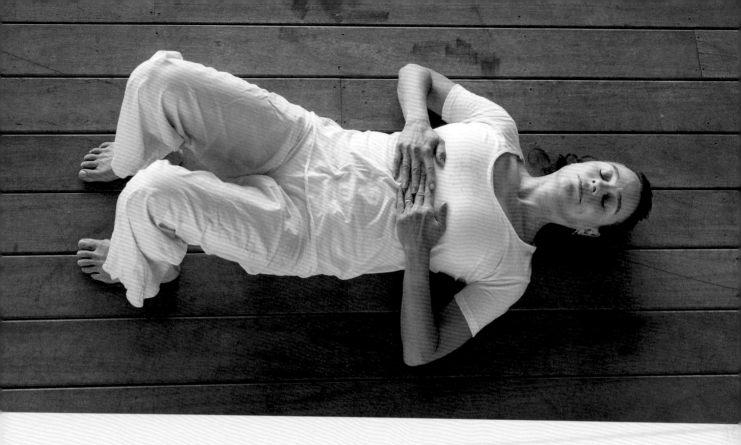

I EXERCISE 2B

Firmly hold the chest down and try to breathe into the belly.

Notice: Is there a difference? Was one type easier or more challenging?

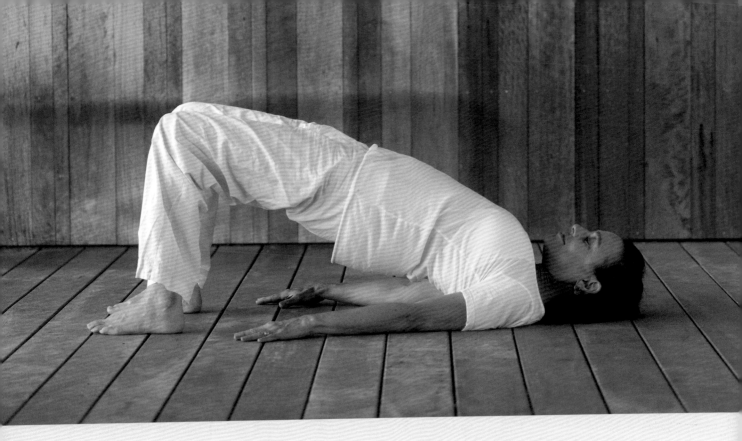

| EXERCISE 3

Begin with natural relaxed breathing (knees bent, feet flat).

Place your hands by your hips, palms facing down.

Lift your hips up towards the ceiling.

Breathe deeply into your belly and notice how easily it rises and falls
in this position.

When you raise your hips like this, it takes the pressure off the
central tendon, especially if that tendon is tight, and enables you to
experience what it's like to take a belly breath.

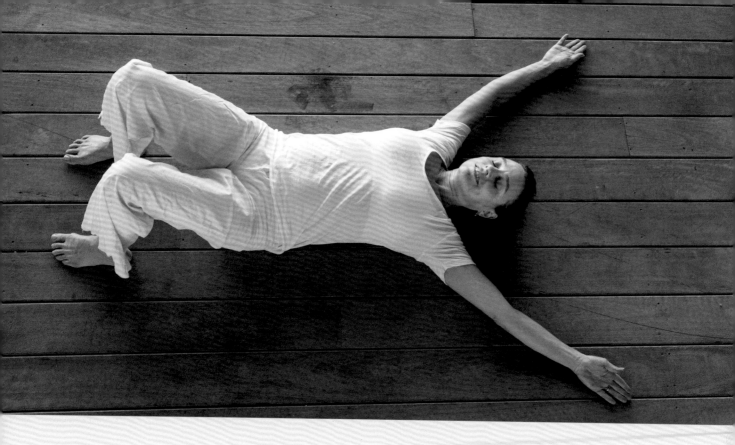

| EXERCISE 4

Begin with natural relaxed breathing (knees bent, feet flat).

Raise your arms over your head and rest the back of your hands on the floor.

Notice: How does this action expand your chest?

On completion of these four exercises, take a moment to reflect on your observations:

Do you find it easy to breathe when you observe your natural relaxed breath?

What feels most natural to you, a chest or a belly breath?

Could you feel the breath in your belly when you raised your hips?

Could you feel the breath in the chest when you raised your arms?

Regardless of what feels better, the ultimate aim is to be able to feel the breath moving naturally between the chest and the belly.

Breathing patterns and the doshas

If you are chest breather, chances are you hold stress in your shoulders and neck and you might have a more sensitive nervous system which can easily lead to an imbalance in Vata dosha.

Chest breathers are also go-getters like our Pitta types and can burn themselves out with too much activity.

If you are a belly breather, chances are you are less reactive and have a robust immune system but you might lack motivation and tend towards depression, which are signs of a Kapha.

In the next section, we'll explore how to do a full complete breath, how to work with ujjayi breath and also learn alternate nostril breathing. Each one of these practices is designed to bring awareness to and expand your breath capacity so that you're in the driver's seat when it comes to your breath.

I Why is breathing properly so beneficial?

Besides the fact that breathing is the one thing we can't do without, deep conscious breathing called diaphragmatic breathing has a ton of benefits.

- It engages the parasympathetic nervous system, which is responsible for calming the heart rate, lowering blood pressure, regulating digestion, elimination and sexual function.

- The steady exchange of oxygen and carbon dioxide feeds the lungs and at the same time clears out toxins.

- It massages the internal organs.

- Breathing through the nose filters the air so that what comes in is free of dust and debris.

- It improves our ability to eliminate waste through the lymphatic system, which has now been discovered to extend all the way into the brain.

- It improves vagal tone.

What's vagal tone?

The vagus nerve is a long cranial nerve, which extends from the brainstem, through the throat, chest and into the abdomen. It plays a major part in keeping our immune system in check. It connects our brainstem to the rest of our body and governs the part of our nervous system that regulates heart rate and gut mobility.

One of the common side effects of diabetes is damage to the vagus nerve, which causes gastroparesis, a delay in emptying food from the stomach.

It doesn't take a textbook definition to understand that if we aren't getting adequate nutrition, our food is fermenting or not absorbing properly, that we're not going to feel great.

Recent studies have observed that low immune function decreases the flow of communication between the brain, the heart and the gut resulting in what's called 'low vagal tone.' In a healthy person, the ability to ward off infections etc is associated with having a high vagal tone. It's been hypothesised that the breathing practices of yoga help to increase vagal tone, thereby boosting the immune system.

| Breathing and the emotions

Another guiding factor in discovering more about the breath is its connection with our emotions. I can vividly remember as a child watching my breath change when I got angry, frightened or sad. When I was happy, I forgot about my breath, but when I wasn't, I felt like my breath turned into a waterfall affecting every muscle and tissue in my body. Places that had been relaxed would contract and I would often curl myself up in ball until the breath returned to normal.

Go back to the image of the upturned mushroom with its spongy stem. Your emotional barometer directly impacts the central tendon of the diaphragm. A shortening of breath tightens that area making it harder to breathe smoothly and deeply.

What's amazing about the breath is it's one of the few functions of the body that can be controlled consciously or unconsciously:

- Unconscious, automatic breath, which continues regardless of whether we think about it or not;

- Conscious breath, where we're aware of the breath and can use it to change our response to any given situation.

When I say 'use it to change your response,' here's a practical example for you. Let's say you test your sugar, it's low, so you freak out. The reaction in your body might look something like this: your heart rate goes up, breathing is agitated and adrenaline is pumping. Taking a few slow deep breaths into the belly while getting what you need to raise your blood sugars can greatly improve the impact that the stress of a low has on your entire system.

One of the best ways to free up your diaphragm is to practice full deep breathing, but what if it's too scary, or you just can't seem to do it? It might not be just the diaphragm that's creating tension. There's another muscle that supports us in freeing and opening the ribcage. It's called the psoas and it's the only muscle that connects the top half of the body to the bottom half. The psoas starts at the lowest vertebrae in the chest (T12) and finishes just inside your hipbone.

A free and flexible psoas means you can easily bend backwards at the hip to achieve hip extension. A backward bending movement also opens the chest and frees the breath. A tight psoas means you are pulled forward (like the motion of being hunched over at your desk) and your hips become accustomed to being 'chair-shaped' or flexed in position. A closed movement like this contracts the chest area and prevents you from breathing freely.

The iliopsoas muscle (another name for the psoas, so-called because it shares an attachment with the iliacus muscle) attaches internally to the lumbar spine and has interconnections with fibres of the diaphragm, which is why it is so extensively affected by the breath. It travels deep in the front of the hip to form an attachment into the femur (thigh) bone. It directly communicates to the nervous system through the surrounding fascia (the connective tissue that surrounds the muscle) as well as via the muscle tissue itself.

A stressful event sends a message from the nervous system to the psoas telling it to contract, which may trigger the fight or flight response. Repeated stressful events can send the psoas into a permanent state of contraction, which hampers our ability to breathe deeply by restricting the natural movement of the lumbar spine where the psoas is attached. This muscle is often a deeply unconscious muscle. Hence, we can be unaware of whether we are experiencing dysfunction in its movement.

Luckily, we can improve the flexibility of the psoas and increase our breath capacity through postures that open the hips and chest.

Let's test the flexibility of your psoas to determine if you'll want to add some psoas stretches to your breathing practice.

First, locate your psoas. Lie on the floor on your back with your knees bent and feet flat on the ground beneath you.

Place your fingertips on the inside of your hipbone and then move in about 1 or 2 inches towards your belly button.

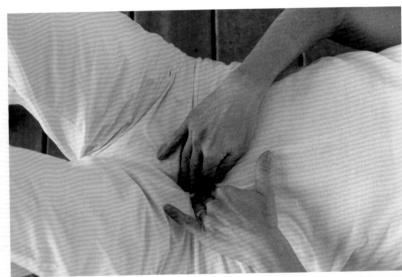

Gently push your fingertips in until you feel a long rope-like tissue.

Lift the corresponding thigh upwards a couple of inches so your foot is just barely off the ground. When you do this, you'll feel the psoas engage.

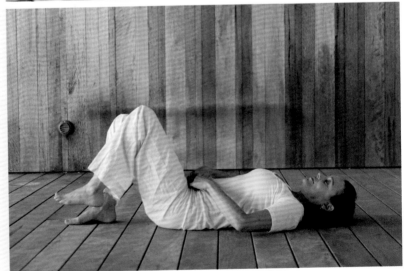

Next, test to see if your psoas is tight.

Lie on a firm table, bench or massage table (your bed will be too soft to do this test) so your buttocks and hips are on the table and your legs are dangling over the edge.

Gently hug one leg in towards your chest while keeping your back flat and your buttocks touching the table. If you hug your knee in too much, your pelvis will scoop under which means the pelvis is no longer in a neutral position.

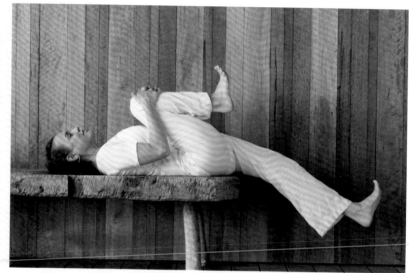

If your hanging leg is hovering in the air and not in contact with the edge of the table, your psoas is tight. If this is the case, you'll want to head over to the modifications section of the book and add the psoas stretches into your routine.

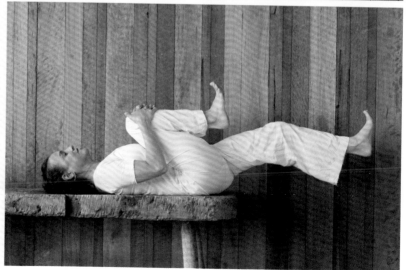

| Muscles that help you breathe better

When I was a kid, I used to laugh when my friends made funny faces, especially when their necks looked like guitar strings. What I didn't know was that these muscles are also involved in the mechanics of breathing. When our breathing is restricted or hampered, the accessory breathing muscles in the shoulders and the neck help out. When we get tense in our neck and shoulders, it's harder to take a deep breath.

Another important muscle that moves without us realising is the pelvic floor. Think of your breath like a wave massaging the spine.

Think of your breath like a wave massaging the spine.

As you breathe in, the spine extends, the ribs expand, the shoulders and collarbones lift and the pelvic floor moves down.

As you breathe out, the pelvic floor lifts, the ribs, shoulders and collarbone relax and the spine returns to the resting position.

The wave of breath moves through extension and gentle flexion, massaging, healing and nourishing your nervous system 24/7.

Holding your breath, forgetting to breathe, being overly identified with emotional states, physical tension and external stressors all contribute to us disconnecting from the breath. Not breathing well or properly limits your body's ability to find balance. Without balance, you don't have the reserves to deal with the everyday details of managing your condition.

Stop...take a moment...and breathe...

You can do this!

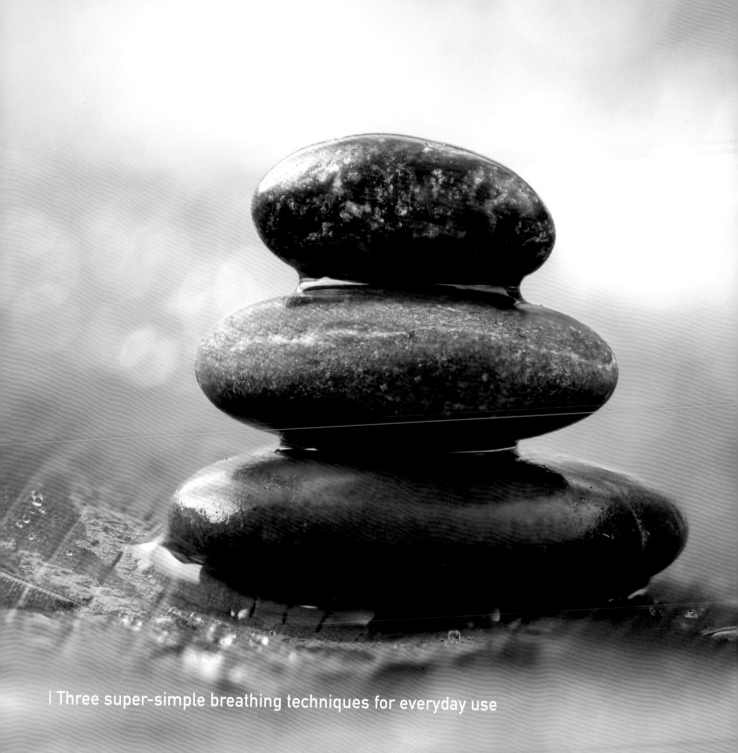

| Three super-simple breathing techniques for everyday use

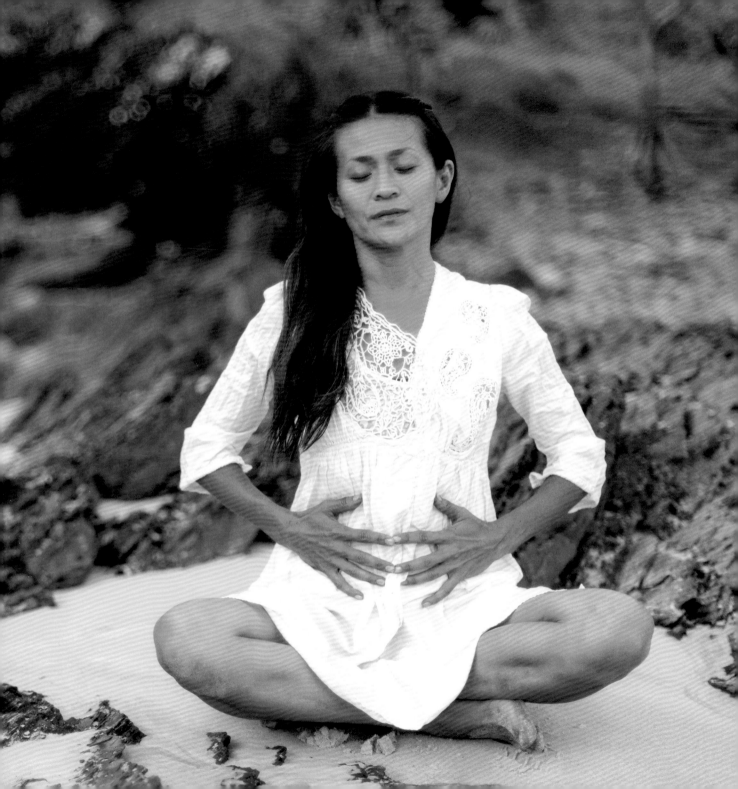

Full complete breath (full yogic breath)

I can't remember how long it took me to master this breath. There was always something to notice in the beginning, especially when I'd had a busy or stressful day. Sometimes my chest was tight or my belly wouldn't relax or I felt super-emotional. Eventually, after doing it regularly for long enough, I fell in love with this breath and now it's a daily practice.

Teaching the body to breathe as fully and completely as possible using both abdominal breathing and chest breathing balances the nervous system. Chest breathing engages the sympathetic nervous system, the energizing part of the system. Abdominal breath activates the parasympathetic nervous system or the relaxed part of the system. Balance between energy and relaxation brings a sense of calm to the body, mind and emotions. Even a few minutes of practice when you first wake up or at the end of the day will remind your body to breathe better in times of stress.

| Technique

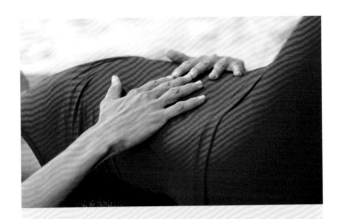

Lie on your back with your knees bent and your feet slightly forward of the hips. Place both hands on the abdomen, tips of the middle fingers touching. Become aware of the breath. Notice the inhale and the exhale.

On the inhalation, expand the abdomen so that the fingers come apart. On the exhalation, feel the abdomen releasing and relaxing, fingers coming together. Repeat this a few times.

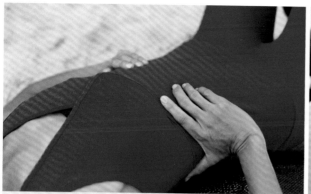
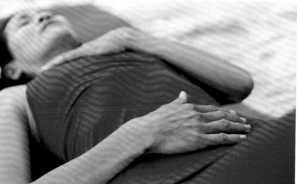

Place your hands on the sides of the ribs. Have your thumbs at the back of the ribcage and your four fingers at the front.

On the inhalation, feel how the sides of the ribs expand and lift. On the exhalation, notice how the ribs come together and the abdomen relaxes as above. Repeat this a few times.

Place one hand on the belly and one hand just below the collarbones.

On the inhalation, feel the abdomen and side ribs expand, and the upper chest and collarbones lift. On the exhalation, feel the abdomen, ribcage and upper chest relax all at the same time. One movement melting into the next. Practice this full complete breath a few times. Then relax and come back to natural relaxed breathing.

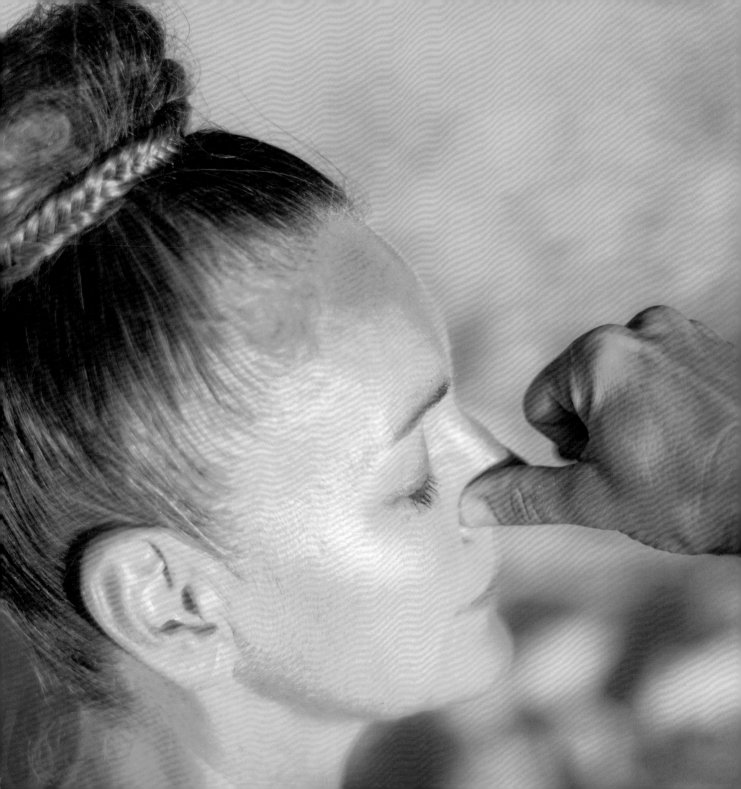

| Alternate nostril breath (nadi shodhana pranayama)

When I first tried this breathing practice, my hands fumbled to hold my nostrils and my arm ached. It took repetition and a relaxed approach to get everything just right. Because this breath balances the right and left hemispheres of the brain, it increased my ability to concentrate, enabling me to be more self-reflective. In yoga, this is called pratyahara (sense withdrawal).

The Alternate Nostril Breath is the ideal breath for balancing the nervous system. This is because it alternates the flow of air through each nostril, and engages the parasympathetic nervous system (the relaxed part of our nervous system and the right hemisphere of the brain) and sympathetic nervous system (the part of nervous system that responds with the fight or flight reflex and the left hemisphere of the brain). As you progress through the repetitions, you'll feel your awareness floating to the corpus callosum, the nerve fibres that join the two sides of the brain. When you aren't dominated by either the left (rational) or right (creative) hemisphere of the brain, you can be with yourself, pure peace and unending stillness.

| Technique

Begin your practice in a comfortable seated position. You can sit on the floor or on a chair. Stay upright with your spine lengthened.

Make a fist with your right hand and extend your thumb, ring finger and little finger.

Make a pincer between your thumb and ring finger. Press your thumb into the soft tissue of your right nostril and press the ring finger into the soft tissue of your left nostril.

Close your right nostril and breathe in through your left nostril.

At the top of your inhalation, close both nostrils and hold the breath briefly.

Release the thumb from the right nostril and exhale out that nostril.

When you reach the bottom of your exhalation, breathe in through the right nostril, hold and block both your nostrils, release the ring finger from the left nostril and breathe out through that nostril.

Continue on your own for at least six more rounds, changing sides at the top of each breath.

To complete your last round, breathe out through the left nostril.

Lower your hand and sit for a few moments, observing the natural flow of breath through both nostrils.

When you're ready, gently open your eyes and take a natural relaxed breath.

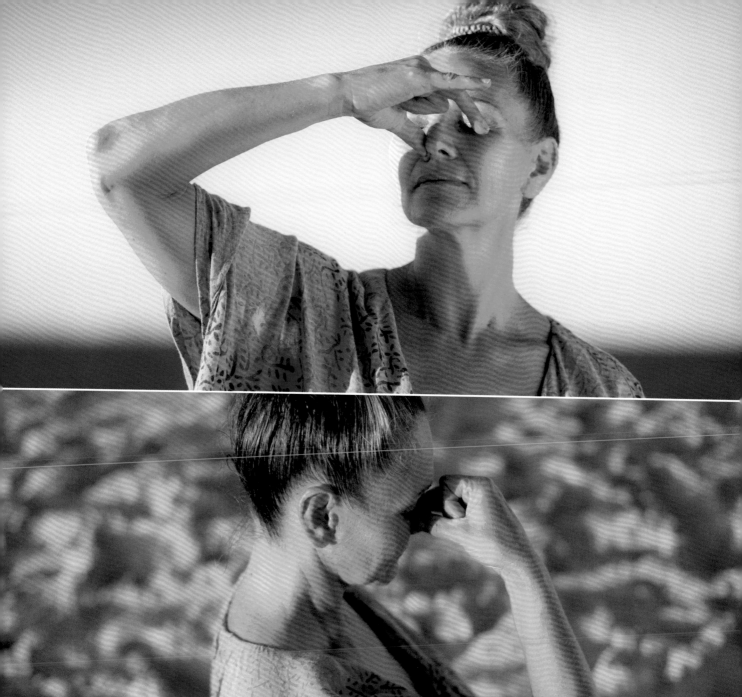

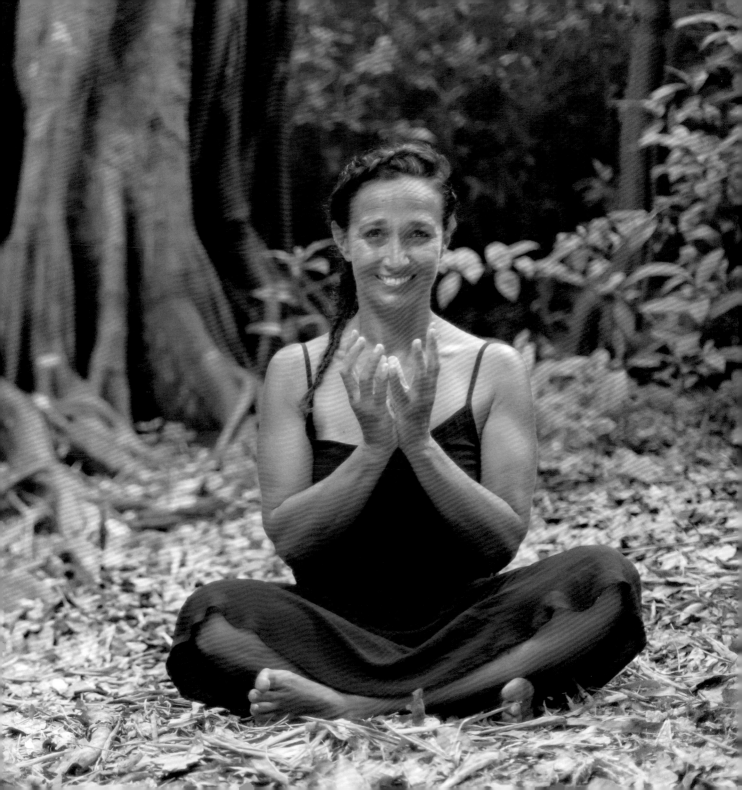

| Ocean breath (ujjayi pranayama)

As an enthusiastic young yogi, I found the ocean breath the most fun. I loved the sensation of closing my throat and feeling the breath lengthen and deepen. Instead of feeling out of breath or overheated in the postures, the ocean breath cooled and calmed me. It gave me a longevity in the pose that I hadn't expected. It was also a touchstone during meditation. Listening to the sound of the breath was like hearing the ocean inside me. It felt purifying, cleansing.

The word ujjayi means victorious, the breath enabling you to build and maintain your stamina during any posture. To practice this technique you make a slight contraction at the back of your throat, like when you make the sound Om or Hum. This makes the breath audible and increases your ability to focus on it while in the posture. Like our other breath practices, ujjayi breathing is calming for the nervous system, and teaches you to deepen and lengthen your breath. Ujjayi is a chest breath and increases the body's ability to absorb prana.

| Technique

Begin your practice in a comfortable seated position. You can sit on the floor or on a chair. Stay upright with your spine lengthened.

Hold your hand in front of your mouth, breathing out onto your palm with your mouth open as if you were fogging up a pair of glasses.

Notice the sound of the breath. It should be audible and breathy like a whisper. Also feel how the throat closes slightly.

Take your hand down, close your mouth and breathe out through your nose making the same whispery sound. The length of your exhalation should increase.

Inhale through your mouth, making the same whispery sound. The breath should feel cool and hit the back of your throat. Think of a minty fresh feeling!

Repeat the same inhalation through the nose with the mouth closed. Try and hear the sound roaring in your ears. Again, the inhalation should take longer than when you were breathing through your mouth.

When you feel confident, inhale and exhale with your mouth closed maintaining ujjayi breath.

You can use this breath throughout your asana practice to help with strength and stamina.

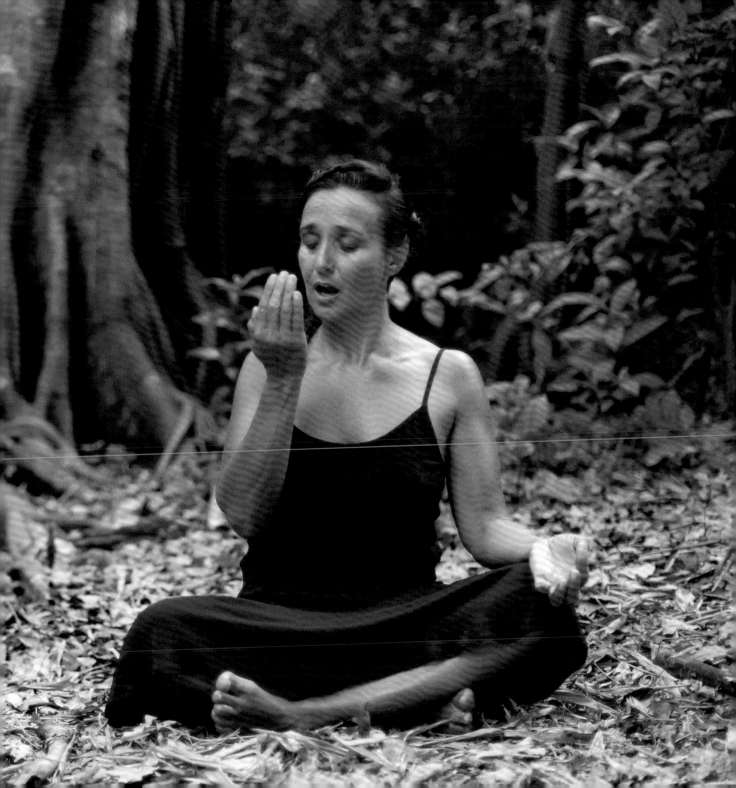

CHAPTER FOUR
ROUTINE

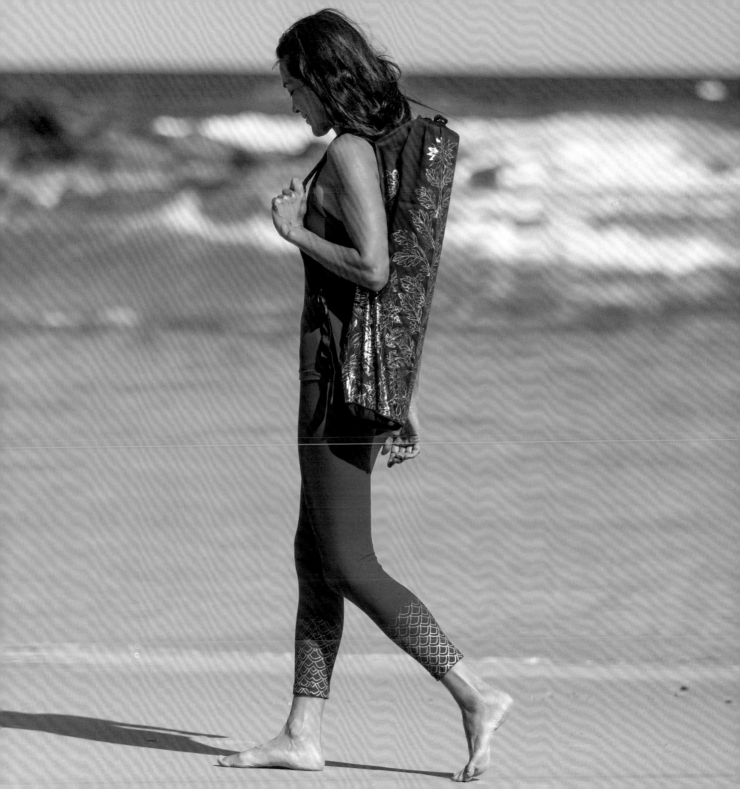

| Regular practice: the need-to-know on medication and exercise

When I was little, I couldn't sit still. I'd twirl, tumble and fall until I was dizzy with glee. When I discovered yoga, I felt like a kid again. The movement created space in my body and space for my breath. The jumbled up things got ironed out; I felt alive and relaxed after every practice.

But then I got sick.

It took me years to accept that physical exercise can either be energizing or draining. It depends on what we power up with. Is your tank full? Or are you starting on empty? Most of us don't even know that we're powering up on an empty tank. We're expected to exercise to manage our weight and keep our insulin levels steady, so we assume that some exercise is better than none. But it's not as straightforward as that.

Understanding your Ayurvedic constitution and how you deal with stress are two considerations you must make when starting a yoga practice. If you're easily stressed, feel ungrounded and lose energy quickly, you may well have depleted your adrenals, as well as working with the disease. Be aware of how your body responds to practice.

If your immune system is running at half-mast, work with a cooling and restorative practice. Any practice that is overly heating or strenuous is only going to make you weaker. Test yourself by watching your breath in every pose. Can you make the breath almost imperceptible, feeling it at the edge of the nostrils? Are you able to keep your mind calm as you execute a posture? The more peaceful you are during the practice, the better you'll feel afterwards. And the more relaxed your nervous system, the easier it is to feel the benefits of the practice in your body.

The sequences that follow are tailored specifically to your current condition (vikruti), but each sequence can also be tailored to your physical, mental and emotional state.

Vata sequence: rejuvenating, strengthening, balancing and rhythmic.

Pitta sequence: cooling, calming, surrendering, stress release, dispersing.

Kapha sequence: invigorating, energetic, enlivening, challenging, opening.

As you monitor your wellbeing before, during and after practice, notice how it feels to do each sequence. Then choose what you feel supports you in that moment. Take your time and practice it as often as possible. Notice what happens. When you feel yourself coming back into what feels like balance for you, you've found the perfect practice.

| Diabetes medication and yoga

Without getting overly technical, it's good to know where you stand when it comes to the relationship between your diabetes medication and exercise. If you have type 2 diabetes, you might be on different types of medication. Before you start the practice, consult with your doctor to find out whether your medication is affected by exercise. A normal yoga practice, although vigorous, doesn't raise the heart rate over 120 bpm. However, if you are overweight, have high blood pressure or a history of heart problems, you will need to take extra care.

If you take insulin, there are certain factors to consider when taking up a yoga practice. Yoga helps to relax the nervous system and increase immune function. Yoga also releases toxins. The type of yoga you choose to practice, the time of day you practice and when you take your insulin can also contribute to whether your blood glucose reading is higher or lower. Understanding your own body and its response to exercise is a good starting point.

Many type 1s have shared with me that they've had hypos during a yoga class. Stopping and dropping a glucose tab or sipping juice can be embarrassing. Plus your yoga teacher may not thoroughly understand the severity of the situation. I have heard of a yoga teacher asking a student to turn down their beeping CGM or take their pump off. You can't expect a yoga teacher to know the ins and outs of diabetes, but I do think they should be respectful and supportive.

In my own experience, I find the less insulin I have on board the less likely I am to have a hypo. So if you've just eaten, bolused for a meal and hit the mat you could be at risk.

One of the best times to practice is in the morning. That's when the liver and endocrine system are producing hormones that naturally raise blood sugar and your body is still burning fat for fuel because you're still in a 'fasted state' before breakfast. As soon as you eat a meal, or even drink cream in your coffee, your body will begin to burn glucose for fuel instead of fat. It's hard to believe, but you should be able to walk for an hour (as long as your basal insulin doses are accurate) without dropping low when you're in a fasted state, first thing in the morning. A 30-minute practice on an empty stomach shouldn't affect your blood sugar. Practicing in the afternoon, however, might because blood sugar tends to be lower at that time of day. When in doubt, you can always experiment lowering your basal dose the night before, turning your pump down 50 percent while you practice, or consuming 15 grams of carbohydrate to keep your blood sugar in a safe range. You may find you need more or less than 15 grams of carbohydrates; everyone's body is different. If you time your snacks with your practice, you don't have to consume additional calories; instead you're just timing your usual food consumption around your exercise appropriately.

Choosing the time of day and type of practice is important. That's why I encourage you to choose a sequence that's right for your type and establish a time of day that works. I get that it's hard to fit yoga into family and work. But think of it like this. With 24 hours in a day, or 1440 minutes, what's a mere 30 minutes? Giving yourself those 30 minutes could be a lifesaver on some days. Especially through those particularly demanding times.

I get that it's hard to fit yoga into family and work. But think of it like this. With 24 hours in a day, or 1440 minutes, what's a mere 30 minutes?

Not only do we live stress-filled lives, but diabetes is well up there on the list of stressful diseases. When we get stressed, the body releases cortisol into the blood stream. Increased cortisol makes you less sensitive to insulin. Reducing stress is key. Believe it or not, even your yoga practice can be stressful, if you place emotional demands on yourself or have high expectations. Approaching your workout with a balanced attitude is more important than mastering the posture.

The beauty of practice is that working the musculature may increase your sensitivity to insulin. Over time, you might find you need less insulin; a great benefit of regular exercise like yoga! No matter how much insulin our bodies need, we still have to be careful about timing our exercise, insulin and nutrition to prevent hypoglycaemia. And according to the experts, it's not just during your yoga practice that you'll need less insulin; the effect may last 12 to 24 hours after any exercise. In short, this means you'll have an overall increased sensitivity to insulin from being active more regularly, as well as a temporary increased sensitivity to insulin after each practice or other exercise.

The different seasons can also affect your insulin requirements. Summer is a much more active season than winter. Spring and autumn tend to be variable. Just like attempting a new pose, you'll have to go slowly when it comes to the different seasons making sure you're moving safely.

As you become familiar with how much the practice impacts your levels, you'll be able to adjust the dose accordingly. The same goes for any weight loss that occurs from taking up a yoga practice. For example, if you are more Kapha and choose a vigorous Vinyasa routine, you may find you lose weight and gain muscle mass which means you'll increase your insulin sensitivity. Even five pounds of weight loss will make a difference.

This applies to dietary changes too. Often when we start a new routine and it's working, we find ourselves wanting to change diet and lifestyle habits as well. Understanding your constitution from an Ayurvedic perspective takes into consideration the types of foods and how they affect you.

If you live with type 2 diabetes, you know that exercise and diet play a huge role in slowing the progression of the disease. You may find it helpful to look at what types of foods aggravate your constitution and what types of foods support you. A lower carbohydrate diet (low glycaemic) may help to improve your glucose control. However, in Ayurveda, grains and legumes are recommended for certain types. It's a fine balance between increasing your insulin sensitivity and eating to your type. But no matter what you do, improving your diet, exercising and decreasing stressors (both mental and physical) can increase your sensitivity to insulin.

Your age will also play a part in the relationship between insulin and exercise. As a young person, in your late teens and early twenties, your body is still maturing, your musculature developing, your hormonal system establishing itself. As an older person, the body loses muscle tone and the joints dry out. As a younger or older woman, the hormones and the liver perform an intimate dance, often increasing the need for insulin. Nothing is predictable or certain. It's nice to approach your practice as you would any new adventure.

| Getting and staying motivated: how to make the practice stick

My step-son has always been an inspiration. He's fascinated with systems of technology and is a pioneer in the field of coding. He's always been brilliant at explaining how systems work, but in his personal life he's struggled with motivation. That is until he discovered meditation. The one thing that kept him coming back and back to the practice was a simple goal-setting exercise at the start. Knowing that he would feel peaceful and focused by the end of the session was his key motivator.

The biggest stumbling block for anyone wanting to take up a new routine is making the practice stick.

So what's the key motivator with practicing yoga to manage your diabetes?

It all depends on you and your constitution, likes and dislikes, and even the type of diabetes you have.

The benefits of yoga practice are:

- Better blood sugar levels

- Increased insulin sensitivity

- Less stress

- Improved fitness

- Balanced mind

- Increased breath capacity

- Weight loss

If you're predominately Vata, though? Your motivators might be increased levels of concentration, an ability to breathe fully and deeply, deep sleep and healthy rest.

If you're predominately Pitta? You might aim for the ability to relax, or stay cool and calm in the face of stress.

And if you're Kapha? You may want to develop your strength, physical and mental, so you can achieve fitness and wellbeing.

Another factor that contributes to motivation is thinking about why you want to start yoga. What will a yoga practice lead you towards? Sometimes the how and the what are no-brainers. I know how to get fit and I know what to do... but why am I doing it?

When you dig deep and ask yourself why you want to try yoga, you might be surprised at what arises as the answer. For me, as a life-long yoga practitioner the why is not just about feeling good or living a long and happy life; it's about acceptance. I get on that mat every day and use my practice to come to terms with what's happened. No matter what my mental or emotional state, yoga returns me to myself.

That's why I do it. Take a moment to think about why you want to do yoga. Write it down or draw a picture. Place it near your mat and when you feel unmotivated look at what you've written. Remind yourself why you're showing up. It will make all the difference!

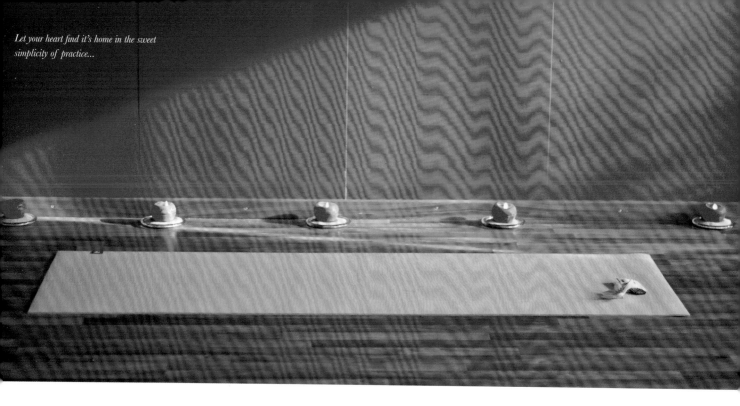

I A Daily Routine

Making a commitment to practice at the same time every day is as important as any other routine in your diabetes management. If you can be consistent in your approach, it will make a huge difference.

Believe it or not, we thrive on routine. Every day the sun rises and sets. As the sun rises, all the birds, animals and plants awaken; as it sets, everything quiets down. Just like different creatures have different sleep and wake cycles, we, according to our constitution, have a personal rhythm. Some of us need more sleep, some less. You might thrive in the morning, but I prefer the evening.

In spite of your personal rhythm, though, the mind loves routine and repetition overall. If you've ever raised a child, you'll see this in action. Give them food, sleep and water at regular intervals and they flourish, just like a plant.

Making a commitment to practice at the same time every day is as important as any other routine in your diabetes management. If you can be consistent in your approach, it will make a huge difference.

I'm such a traveller. It's normal for me to cross time zones more than three times a year. When that happens, having a routine has been an absolute lifesaver. Knowing that morning is my practice time means I make that effort to roll out my mat in the hotel, the AirBnB, the cabin, wherever! And go for it. I always feel refreshed after practice no matter how jet-lagged I am.

The time of day you practice is important but so is place. I like to think of it like Pavlov's dog, if you know that experiment. Here's a reminder, just in case you don't. Pavlov would ring a bell every time he brought the dog food and the dog would salivate. Over time the dog learned to associate the sound of the bell with food, so when Pavlov rung the bell but didn't bring the food, the dog would salivate anyway.

Okay, so give me some license here.

Having a specific space to practice is like that. If you leave your yoga practice space set up, mat rolled out, some beautiful items to gaze at, comfy blankets and props. You'll associate the space with the desired goals you've set for yourself and you'll keep heading back for more.

One of the best gifts you can give yourself is a space you feel at home in. Speaking with other friends who have diabetes, there's a general consensus that food, although necessary, is kind of annoying. One friend mentioned that if he didn't have to eat he wouldn't. I feel the same. For me, a clean open yoga space is my chocolate bar. It fills me up. Having diabetes means I enjoy things that people without diabetes might take for granted. It's not my choice exactly, but it helps me to accept what is.

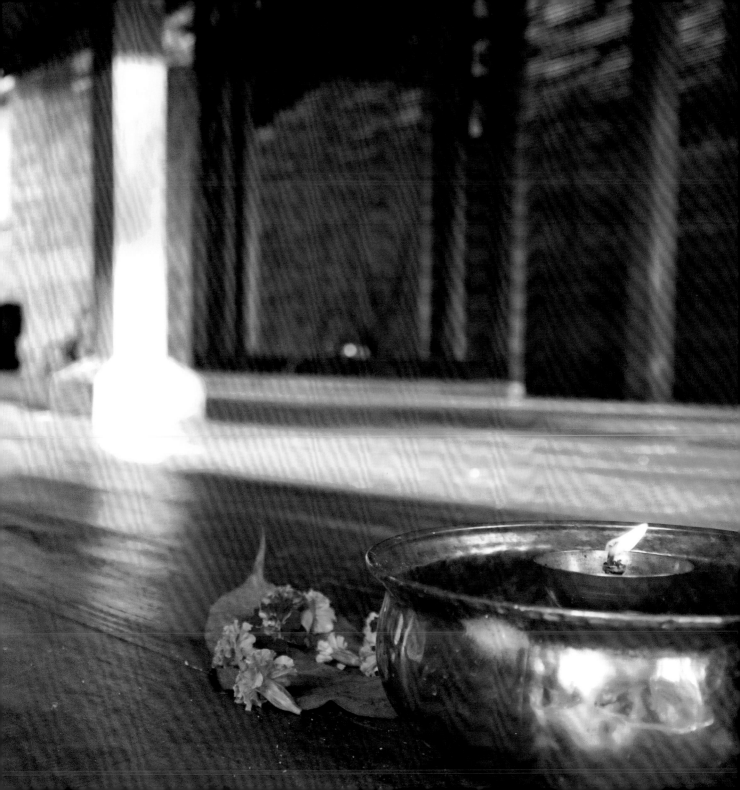

CHAPTER FIVE
CONTEMPLATION

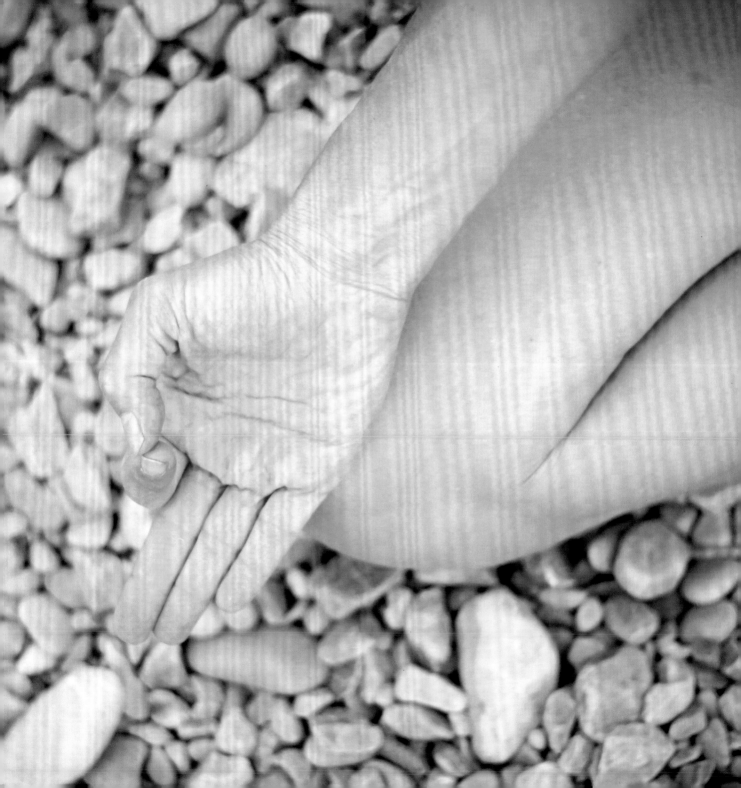

| The worst meditator

Everyone has their own way of getting quiet. Mine will be different to yours. When I talk of 'getting quiet,' I don't mean peace and quiet free from noise; I mean that feeling you get when you catch yourself daydreaming, lost in the thought of a cloud or whatever. Not quite asleep but totally relaxed.

Another way of expressing this is by calling it 'mindfulness', which is just a fancy word for meditation. Do you think of meditation as a state of attainment? Have you already given up on yourself because you know without a doubt you'll never ever be able to do it?

I don't tell many people this but I was the worst meditator ever when I started out. As soon as I tried to count my breaths or observe sensations in my body, my mind would whirl at a 100 million miles an hour.

I don't tell many people this but I was the worst meditator ever when I started out. As soon as I tried to count my breaths or observe sensations in my body, my mind would whirl at a 100 million miles an hour. And I'd get super-creative and have another million ideas. I couldn't see the point in slowing down my thought process when I was coming up with the next Michelangelo. I wasn't convinced that meditation worked until I met my friend Louisa. The only reason I tried it was because she said it would be fun to bunk together in a dome on a hippie farm while meditating with a former Burmese monk who looked like a rock star. Hmm, I was sceptical. Did I have the best time? Not exactly. Did I learn how to sit still and observe my thoughts? Well, it was a start.

Fast forward to my trip to the Blue Mountains. I swapped my car keys and wallet for a silent Vipassana retreat. Crazy me, I'd signed up for 11 hours of meditation a day for 10 days straight. No talking, minimal eating, no writing, reading or yoga. (Although I snuck in a yoga pose or two in the bathroom stalls when no one was looking.)

By day 3, I was able to watch my breath like a pro. Day 6, and I was exploring altered states. And by day 10? I'm like a kid on crack. Everything jumped out at me in technicolor. Leaves had never looked so green. Food had never tasted so good. But perhaps, if you put anyone on a starvation diet, deprive them of their technology and keep them from talking, they'd get carried away when they got out too.

I was so passionate after that first retreat that I started meditating every day twice a day. I kept that up for years until I realized it was going nowhere. The practice wasn't actually helping me cope with my life. It was acting like a temporary tranquillizer. But as soon as I stopped meditating all the anxiety and tension would flood back in.

I So why the change?

I got divorced, my son left home, I sold my house and went on an extended trip to India. While there, I was fortunate enough to study traditional knowledge not readily available to those of us in the West. Some of those studies had to do with understanding what meditation is and what it's not.

Here's what I've come to understand.

Meditation is NOT:

a state
a practice
stopping the thoughts
enlightenment
a means to an end

Meditation IS:

concentration
effortless
happening in every moment
interchangeable with the words 'peace', 'yoga', 'stillness'
oneself

So after establishing what meditation is, what happens next? Why do it? How do you do it? And will you ever manage to know yourself as that effortless presence?

This is where it gets really cool. You can never know yourself as this or that. You can only ever be yourself.

| Changing meditation to concentration

So let's flip our understanding of the word meditation and refer instead to concentration. In yoga, it's called dharana. Dharana is focussing the mind in on one point for an extended period of time. When you do that, it takes the mind out of its preoccupation with a thought. Remember the story of the boy who made the wish-fulfilling monkey run up and down the pole and it saved his life? For any one of us, it's easy to concentrate when we're absorbed in a task. How quickly does time pass when you're doing what you love? Concentration as a practice is exactly the same.

The mind, if given the right technique, becomes laser-focused. All the juicy benefits associated with meditation kick in at that point. Those might be:

Less stress
Better sleep
More energy
Increased focus
Improved digestion
Lower blood pressure

And numerous other benefits.

It's all about having the right kind of concentration practice for you. I might be more visual whereas you might be auditory and your friend might be different again and prefer kinaesthetic techniques. The way you learn determines the way you practice. This is where I absolutely love the diversity of yoga. The different elements of practice relate to each person and their ability to process sensory input.

In relationship to chronic illness and chronic stress, having a solid dharana practice is a key component. Most people think, to meditate/concentrate, they'll need to be able to watch their mind or stop their thoughts. None of those are a requirement for the practice. All that's required is an intention to let go of the thoughts while performing a repetitive activity like: watching your breath, repeating a sound, or visualizing an image.

A concentration practice requires your complete attention. Closing your eyes, tuning out the outside world, closing the mouth and sitting still is like shutting all the windows and doors in your home in the evening. If you keep your eyes, ears and mouth open, the external world is still getting a foothold. Closing the apertures of the senses signals to the mind that you are sitting quietly.

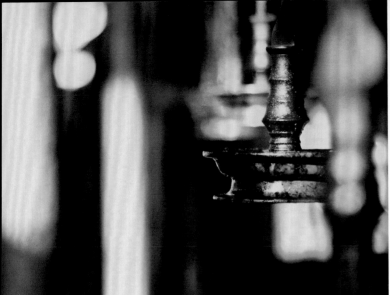
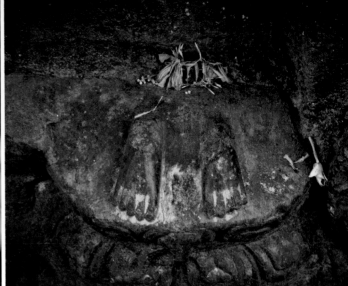

The flame of awareness can
never be extinguished...

I Meditation in the context of the word YOGA

Like meditation, the word 'yoga' is also misunderstood. In the West, we have learned that yoga means union or to yoke and that we're yoking (uniting) the mind to the breath, the body to the mind. We're also told that we're joining with our spirit or soul. I used to think that when I meditated I was plugging into some sort of universal socket and getting super-charged with spiritual energy. Now my goal is to demystify all the different aspects of yogic life. Starting with the meaning of yoga.

Yoga means oneness. One without a second. Wholeness.

How can something that is already whole need to be united or joined? It just doesn't make sense. The word yoga says it all: already whole and complete, there is nothing you need to do to be that. Any practice is just there to remind you of what you already are. So meditation/ concentration is the practical tool we employ to remember ourselves.

I Concentration: Which practice suits you

For this book, I've chosen three different kinds of practices specific to the doshas. But that doesn't mean if you are a Kapha type you can only do the Kapha practice. Try each one on for size over a two-week period. Give it enough time to see if it resonates with you. Once you've chosen your favorite, stick with it for 40 days. That's how long it takes for a practice to truly release all the goodies.

Does 40 days of concentration sound scary? Don't panic! I started practicing in baby steps. One day at a time.

I love what my teacher Alan Finger used to say.

Start with just 5 minutes. As you get used to the feeling, aim for 10, then 15, and eventually 20. By the time you get to 20, you'll want to sit for 40 and then you'll never want to stop.

(I found it handy to use a timer to keep up with how long I was sitting.)

I How to get comfortable

Before I share any of the techniques, it's important that you are comfortable while you practice. If you've got a stabbing pain in your back, for example, you definitely won't want to do it. The best way to find out what's comfortable is to try a few different ways of sitting.

1. Sit in a chair

2. Cross-legged seat (check that your knees are slightly lower than your hips and if they aren't you'll need to elevate your buttocks on a blanket)

3. Straddle a bolster

4. Sit against a wall for back support

| The Sunrise meditation for vata

As a creative and visionary type, colorful visual techniques work well to occupy your mind. During the practice, you'll visualize the three colors we see in the sky as the sun is rising. Blue, rose and gold. At that time of day, the earth is in transition, the animals are quiet and prana is at its most potent. It's the perfect time of day, not only to calm the mind but to absorb energy into the body.

To begin, set an intention for the practice. It could be anything. Start with something simple like "I want to feel calm at the end of the practice." It could also be something more personal like "I dedicate this practice to achieving more balanced blood sugars." It doesn't really matter what the intention is. What matters is that you set it. Once a goal (intention) is in play, the mind and body enjoy working towards its achievement. As we covered in the earlier chapter on thoughts, every thought has a desired outcome and the thought will keep traveling until it reaches its destination.

The Sunrise Meditation combines color and breath to heal and nourish your system.

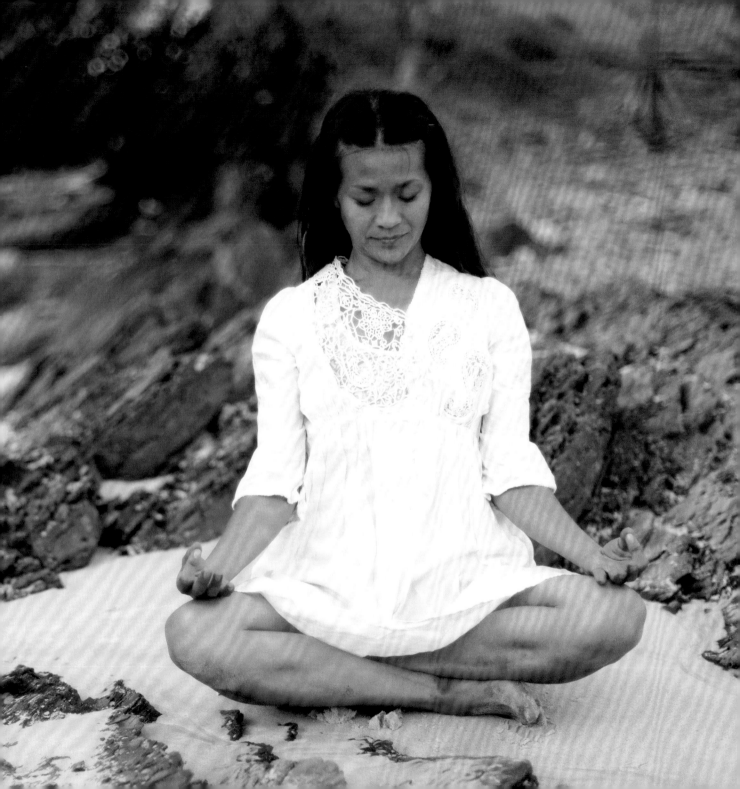

| Technique

Exhale all the air out of the body (through the nose) slightly squeezing the throat muscles to do so.

Breathe in through the nose for a count of four visualizing that you're breathing in blue sky-colored light from your toes all the way to the crown of your head.

Drop the chin slightly, as if you were holding an orange under it, and hold the breath for a count of four, visualizing a pink rose mist swirling into every cell of the body.

Exhale through the nose for a count of four, imagining a golden light surrounding your entire body in an egg shape.

Repeat for 3 to 5 minutes or as comfortable.

When you are ready, gently open your eyes and head into your day.

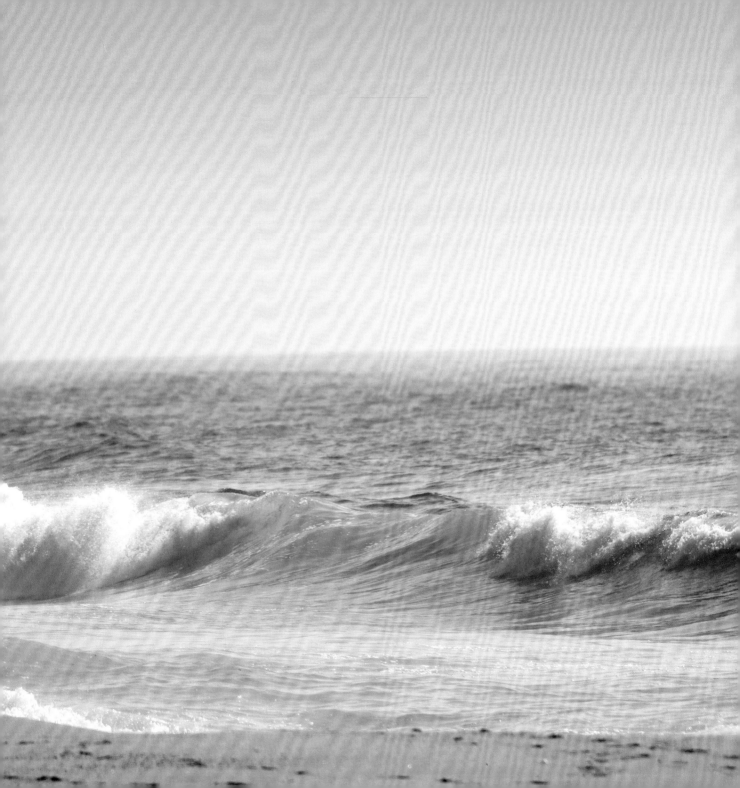

| The Soham meditation for pitta

As a fiery type, the act of trying to concentrate can often incite frustration. To balance that Pitta, we need to counteract that fire. And what counteracts fire? Water.

The sound of the ocean is like the sound of the breath when you cover your ears and listen carefully. To balance Pitta, you'll be using sound (mantra) to focus your mind. One of the most profound mantras is the natural sound the breath makes as we breathe in and out. This is happening automatically 24,600 or so times a day. If you place your hands over your ears and breathe in, you'll hear the sound So. Keeping your hands over your ears when you breathe out, you'll hear the sound Ham.

The Soham Meditation is an ancient technique that works effectively to calm and cool the nervous system and mind.

Again, set an intention for your practice. It could be anything, something simple like "I want to feel relaxed at the end of the practice" or more personal like "I dedicate this practice to accepting things as they are."

| Technique

Engage ujjayi breath. Long slow inhalation, long slow exhalation.

Feel the breath become even. Even count for inhalation, even count for exhalation. Continue counting the breath.

Move the awareness to the pelvic floor, sensing the space between the pubic bone and the tailbone.

On your next inhalation, for an even count, visualize the breath flowing up the center of the spine to the middle of the brain.

On the next exhalation, for an even count, visualize the breath flowing down the center of the spine. Continue like this for as long as is comfortable.

Add the sound (mantra) So on the inhalation and Ham on the exhalation.

Chant the mantra internally to yourself.

Keep breathing in the sound So and breathing out the sound Ham for about 3 to 5 minutes or as comfortable.

When you're ready, gently open your eyes and head into your day.

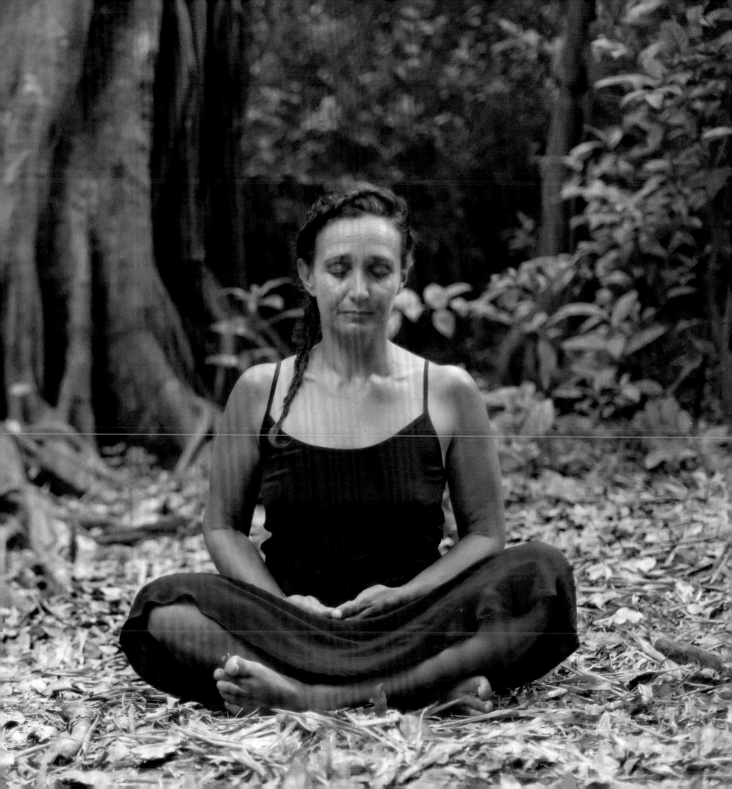

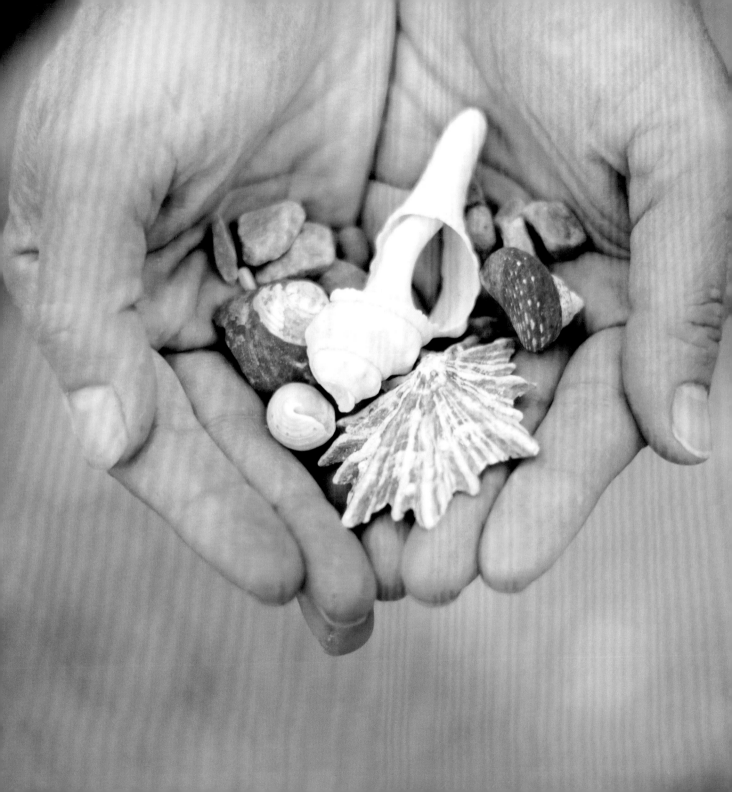

I The Satyam meditation for kapha

As a loving and patient type, you don't struggle as much to sit still as the other doshas. But that doesn't mean meditation isn't a powerful tool in your toolkit. Kaphas struggle with letting go or getting stuck in thoughts that lead to lethargy and depression. For you, letting go of limiting emotions is key.

The word Satyam means truth. Truth ever present as yourself. When you break the word in two you get Sat, which means ever-existing, and Yam. Yam is a sound which relates to the element of air, being light and subtle, as opposed to the heaviness of the earth and water elements. The practice moves from the gross to the subtle, starting with breath and movement, colorful imagery and finally sound.

Movement, breath and sound are a wonderful way for you to perfect your ability to concentrate and stay stimulated.

During the practice we will also be working with a mudra. Mudras are specific hand gestures which naturally calm and balance the nervous system. When you hold a mudra you join specific fingers together, i.e. the thumb and forefinger to form a complete circle or all the fingers together into a prayer position like when we say Namaste. For our practice we will be working with the lotus mudra, called padma mudra.

As with all the meditations, set an intention for your practice. It could be anything, maybe starting simply with "I want more energy" or something more personal like "I dedicate this practice to letting go of grief."

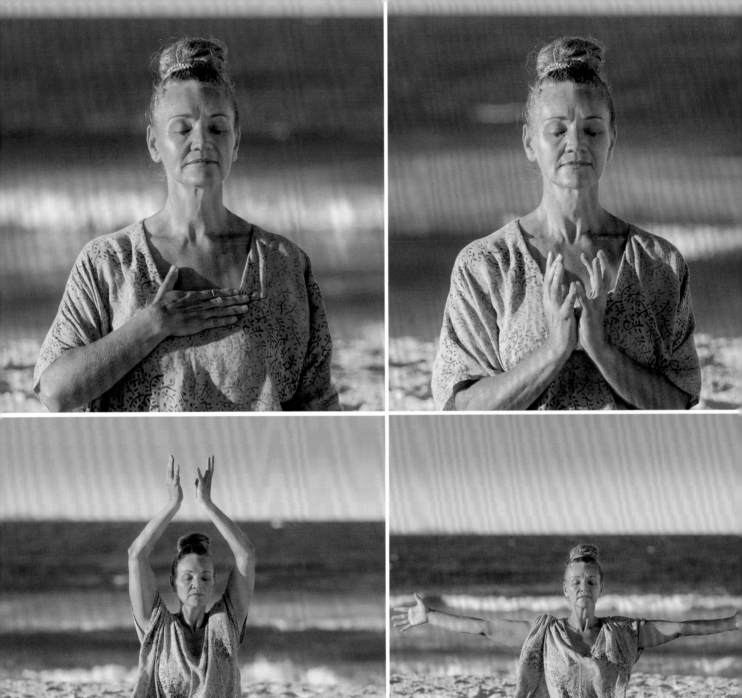

| Technique

Place your hand on your heart. Feel the warmth of your hand at your heart and notice your breath. Take a few moments here to let the mind settle.

Bring the heels of your hands together and extend the fingers so your hands are in the shape of a cup or lotus (padma mudra).

Imagine that inside your cup/lotus are all the emotions and feelings that haunt you. Don't think too hard about it. See what arises.

As you inhale, lift the cup/lotus by straightening your arms sending the emotions back to pure unconditioned awareness.

As you exhale, open your arms to the side and surround yourself in a fine purple mist.

Repeat this a few times, lifting the cup/lotus overhead on inhalation, surrounding yourself with a fine purple mist on exhalation.

Repeat the moving meditation a few more times silently adding the sound Sat on inhalation and Yam on exhalation.

Let go of the movement with the arms, resting the hands on the thighs.

Continue to chant internally: Sat as you feel the breath moving up the spine to the crown of the head on inhalation; Yam surrounding yourself in the fine purple mist on exhalation. Think of it like an internal fountain replenishing itself with every in and out breath.

Finally, feel the sound Satyam resting like a pulse at the center of your heart. Rest there for another few moments.

When you're ready, gently open your eyes and head into your day.

CHAPTER SIX
SETTING UP YOUR PRACTICE SPACE

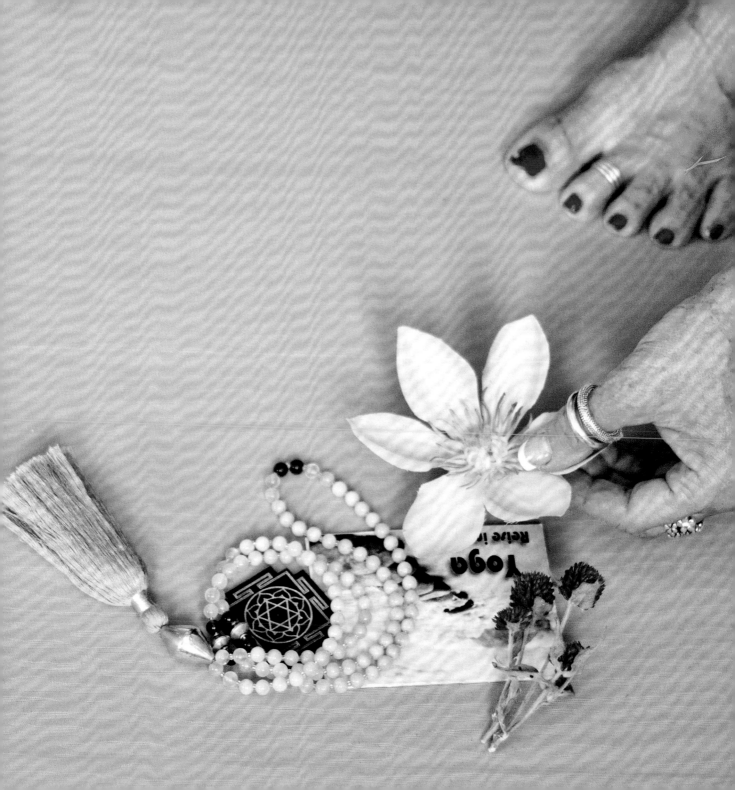

| Setting up your practice space

Over the years, my personal practice space has changed many times over. When I first started, I was living in a tiny cabin in a place called Mullumbimby in northern New South Wales, Australia. I would practice in the living room facing our local mountain. I didn't light candles or incense and knew nothing about the Hindu deities. In those days, our yoga mats were from the local car manufacturer. We'd use the non-ribbed side of the rubber matting they use under your feet in cars to roll out for our practice. Blocks were handmade and wooden. Blankets came from the local army-navy store. And belts were flown in from a yoga school in India. I also put up a rope in a loop on the veranda so I could climb into it and hang upside down.

To be honest, not much has changed for me. I did go through a phase where my practice space transformed into a place of gratitude and devotion, filled with flowers, soothing images and candles etc, but ultimately having all that stuff is irrelevant. What serves me best is a simple clear space, with natural light and open windows.

Choosing a place to practice every day is important because you want it to be a haven, a place to come back to yourself. Sure, you can roll out the mat amidst the kids, dogs and dinner. But I would encourage you to find a space where you can be private, relaxed and feel nurtured.

Some people find a spot in their bedroom, perhaps at the foot of the bed, facing a favorite painting or window. You might carve out a corner in your home office, or enjoy practicing on the back patio in the garden away from the elements. Once you choose the space, be consistent. Let your family know this is your place for yoga. Keep it uncluttered and bring things to the space that remind you of beauty, peace, stillness and love. Whatever you feel you need to make it your happy place, do it!

I Indoor versus outdoor practice

Depending on the time of day, location and your constitution, you may wonder whether you should practice inside or outside. My partner and I have tried it all. We lived in India and Bali for a few months out of the year and it was way more convenient and cooler to practice outside in the early morning or early evening. At those times, the prana is closer to the earth and more easily absorbed by the body.

If you want to practice outside, make sure you never practice in the wind or direct sunlight. You'll want to find somewhere sheltered from the elements, otherwise you'll increase both the Vata and Pitta in your system. It's happened to me on a number of occasions and I've had to learn the hard way. If you choose to practice inside, make sure you're not practicing in direct sunlight there either, but do practice near an open window. If you're in a hotel room with sealed windows, you might want to turn off the air-conditioning or make sure it's not directly blowing on you.

I The best props and tools

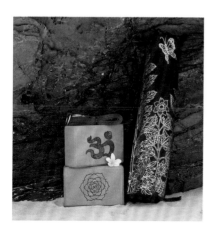

People often ask me what the best tools are for the practice, what kinds of mats, blocks, blankets and straps you need to use, what you wear.

The truth? Most mornings I roll out of bed onto a thin travel mat and practice in my PJs. It's not about what I wear or what sort of mat I have. I couldn't care less to be honest. However, as a new practitioner, it's handy to have a mat with good grip, that feels right under your hands and feet, and that isn't toxic. Expensive yoga mats are not necessarily better mats. In order to find the best mat for you, ask yourself the following questions. Then do some online research and choose accordingly.

Do I sweat a lot in the practice?

Am I sensitive to rubber, PVC, or other materials?

Is being ecologically responsible important to me?

Is price an issue?

Do I want something thick and sturdy that lasts, or lightweight because I'm on the go?

Does my height make a difference to the size of the mat, because I'm tall/short?

Once you've chosen your mat, you might like to purchase a mat bag so it stays dust-free. It's also much nicer to use your own mat at the studio or gym because it's more hygienic for you.

Other useful props are foam or cork blocks (to bring the floor towards you for some postures); a cotton strap (if you can't easily reach your toes in seated and standing balancing poses); a bolster for restorative postures; a yoga blanket to make your seated position more comfortable.

However, if you want to keep things simple the following replacements will do just fine:

- For blocks, use two thick books or two tightly rolled up towels

- For a strap, use a long belt, sash or lightweight sarong

- As a bolster, a few pillows stacked on top of one another, sofa cushions or thick towels rolled into a sausage shape

- As a yoga blanket, a thick folded towel, throw cushions, regular bed blanket

I What to wear for yoga

I already mentioned PJs, but just in case you're wondering if you should invest in the latest branded yogawear, I would suggest the following:

Tight yoga clothes restrict airflow. Loose comfortable clothes allow for freedom of movement. Choose something warmer for winter and cooler for summer. Cotton fabrics are best especially if you sweat a lot. If you want to be able to see your alignment, choose cotton leggings and a more closely fitting top.

Generally, the more freedom you have when you move, the more relaxed you'll be. For the purposes of seeing the postures, the models in the sequences in this book are wearing tightly fitting, specifically designed yoga clothes. For your own practice, however, anything you feel good in will be perfect. We've got enough on our plate without having to worry about how we look on the mat in our own home.

If you'd like to know more about where to get yoga props and clothes, head to the resources section at the back of the book.

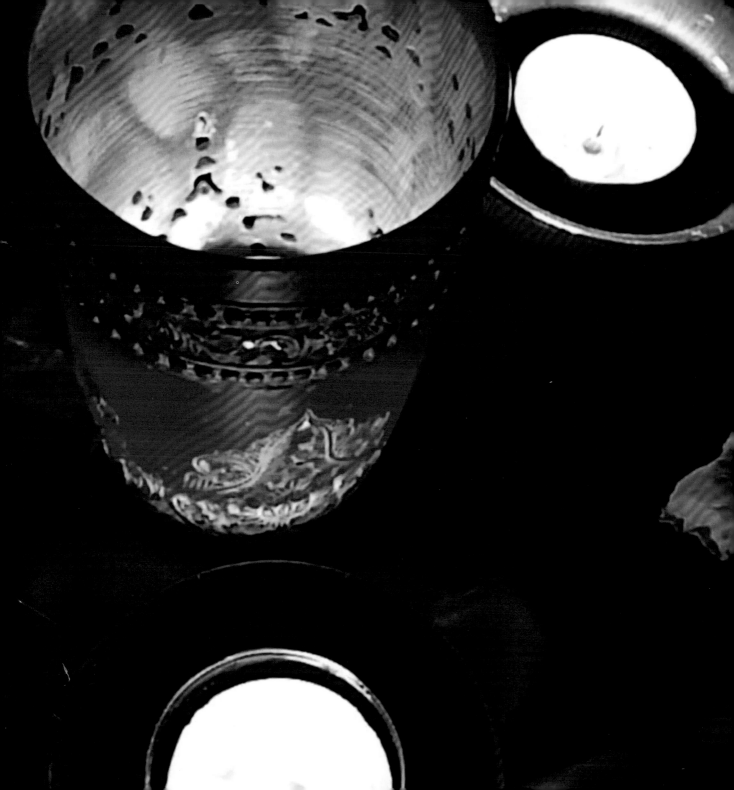

I Creating beauty in your yoga space

Finally, a note on creativity and devotion. As I deepened my practice and faced the reality of having diabetes, I felt I wanted to surround myself with reminders to let go, soften and refine my emotional attitude. Bringing in flowers, lighting a candle, burning some essential oils and playing soothing music helped me to surrender and accept my diagnosis. It wasn't something I did naturally. It grew on me and I found that the creation of beauty in my designated yoga space developed different aspects of my creativity. I became a designer, an artist and a florist. There were days where there was so many photos, drawings, flowers and statues crowded onto my altar that my eye, not knowing where to fall, turned inwards. On other days, a solitary candle and a photo of my mother opened the floodgates.

Making an altar is an extremely simple and powerful tool for keeping your yoga practice fresh and inspired.

Making an altar is an extremely simple and powerful tool for keeping your yoga practice fresh and inspired. If you'd like to create one, here are a few ideas to guide you:

- Practice where you can see your altar

- Create your altar on a low table, the floor, your dresser, anywhere really. All you need is a flat surface to place items

- Think about images, statues, items that hold meaning for you and gather them together; a photo of a loved one, a rock or shell you've collected, a beautiful ring or necklace, feathers, cards

- Pick or buy your favorite flowers and select a candle that you can relight or use tea lights

- Choose a scented oil for your oil burner or light your favorite incense

- Choose a beloved fabric to cover your chosen surface

- Put on some music and go to town; draping the cloth, arranging the photos and mementos, placing flowers down

Start each practice with an intention or dedication. It could be for yourself or someone else. Something that matters to you personally or globally.

As you create the altar, think about your vision for yourself and your diabetes management. What would you like to change? What can you commit to? How do you see yourself in 3, 6 or 12 months time? Think about loved ones. Feel grateful.

Once the altar is complete, sit or stand in front of it and take it all in. Let it speak to you.

You can update the altar on a daily basis, removing old flowers, relighting a candle, or you can leave it as is. For me, the altar is a touchstone. Once it's there, I feel like I've come home. It's perfect for the Pitta in me as it speaks to my devotional heart.

If you don't have the inclination to create an external altar, an internal one is just as good. Start each practice with an intention or dedication. It could be for yourself or someone else. Something that matters to you personally or globally. Each of the sequences in the book starts with an intention. Let this be a starting point for your own visions and aspirations.

Because in the end, your heart is the best altar.

| Daily nurturing routine

Dinacharya for diabetes

Something shifted for me when I realized that I had to take extra care of myself. I began to notice how I structured my day with regards to eating, exercising, working, playing and sleeping. Rather than just doing everything sporadically, I had to reinvigorate the part of me that, as a young teenager, was disciplined enough to attend hours of ballet classes, do her homework and get to bed at a reasonable hour.

In Ayurveda, having a regular routine is called dinacharya. Dinacharya isn't just doing certain tasks at a certain time each day. It's implementing self-care practices that can make a difference to your stress levels and help manage your diabetes. At the core of your daily self-care routine is your yoga practice.

Rather than bombard you with a host of to-dos, here are four simple rituals I stick to every single day, which have made a huge difference to my overall attitude and wellbeing.

1. Wake up before the sun rises and greet the day with gratitude. Rising before the sun means you will have more energy available to you throughout the day. At dawn, the prana is still low in the atmosphere and easily absorbed by the body. Perfect for type 1s who need to build energy. For type 2s, it's a great time for dynamic breathing or a walk in nature or along the beach.

2. Sip hot water instead of tea throughout the day. Plain hot water is cleansing and eliminates toxins. It's also warming and nurturing. For type 1s, it lubricates and soothes the nervous system; for type 2s, it eliminates accumulated waste.

3. Give yourself a nurturing head and foot massage before bed. No matter what your type, massaging the feet before bed balances the nervous system and promotes sound sleep. In Ayurveda, specific oils are used depending on your constitution. But to keep it simple any plain massage oil or cream to keep your feet soft will work, especially if you suffer from skin cracks or nerve damage. Make sure to massage the whole foot focusing on the pads of the feet, around the heel and Achilles tendon, and between the toes.

4. Yoga nidra is a phrase to describe a deep and conscious state of rest. Unlike the corpse pose, you stay alert while relaxing different parts of the body, counting breaths and sensing and visualizing various physical and emotional states.

Benefits of yoga nidra are akin to going into a deep sleep. Our brain has the capacity to work in different states of awareness: waking state, relaxed state, dream state and deep sleep state. There is also a fifth state called the gamma state, which happens at the point of orgasm or during any ecstatic activity. Even though science has categorized these states as separate to each other, in reality they're all happening at once. We choose where to place our attention. For instance, when you're hard at work nutting out a problem or completing a task you're in the beta brainwave state. If you decide to take a break, watch TV or read a book, you can become so relaxed you're nearly asleep. That's the alpha wave. The alpha wave quite naturally takes you into the dream state which is the theta wave. Before you know it, you're out for the count. This is the delta wave. Everything disappears. No thoughts, no ideas, no individuality, no problems. Bliss.

The theory behind yoga nidra is that as you are led through a series of steps, starting with relaxing different parts of the body, observing the breath and finally working with visualization, quite naturally you flow into the alpha wave, which relaxes the nervous system and reduces your stress.

You can either incorporate all four of these practices into your daily routine or choose one according to your specific needs. I recommend beginning slowly and simply. Less is more. I've always found that when I try to do everything at once it's easy to give up. I encourage you to make your practice sustainable. That's when you'll get the best results.

At the end of this section, there are guidelines on how to choose the perfect practice for your type. You'll also find a practice chart outlining how the sequences, breathing and meditation techniques and daily routines all work together. You'll find the yoga nidra after the last dosha sequence.

And a final note for those really tough days...

One of the biggest challenges in my life has been to deal with my anger. Even when I was small, the feeling of frustration would well up in me to the point where I just felt so alone and incapable that I wanted to scream. These feelings haven't gone away just because I took up yoga. When I was diagnosed, I felt so defeated. I couldn't understand why this had happened to me. I'd spent my life doing everything right. Or had I?

I tried to find a reason why...was it because I shoplifted as a tween? Was it the time I got kicked out of ninth grade for hanging out with the wrong crowd or because I kicked that door in at high school and never owned up?

In a way, I wish it were that simple. Equating a bad action with a bad result. But as I've grown up, I've learned that life doesn't work like that. No one out there is judging me for anything I've ever done. Yes, I made choices and am dealing with the consequences. But there are some things we can't control and can't expect. Like my mother dying, or being in New York City on 9/11, or hearing my diagnosis. Significant parts of my life that no one could have altered.

| On gratitude and the power of devotion…

This is where gratitude comes in. Gratitude is one of those tools you can use anywhere anytime when the going gets tough.

Even before my diagnosis, I had a gratitude diary and made a list each night of all the good things that had happened that day. It softened those feelings of frustration and anger, and helped me to see that I had so much to be thankful for. I still practice being grateful on a daily basis, but now it's been woven into my yoga practice too. It's become devotional, a moment of quiet, a chance to reflect.

Even before my diagnosis, I had a gratitude diary and made a list each night of all the good things that had happened that day…

There's lots of fancy terms these days for working with gratitude, but I want to offer you something simple. Something that you can do just before you start the practice and something you can bring in at the very end.

Once you're settled on your mat, bring the palms of your hands together right at the center of your heart. Take a moment and watch your breath as it enters and leaves the nostrils. Then think of someone you love, something that brings you peace, or a place you feel at home. Feel your gratitude. Let the words and images flood in. It needn't take more than a few seconds to remember the grace of your existence. Your ability to be right here right now, alive, experiencing creation, what a gift! Without you, none of this would exist.

You are the meaning in everything.

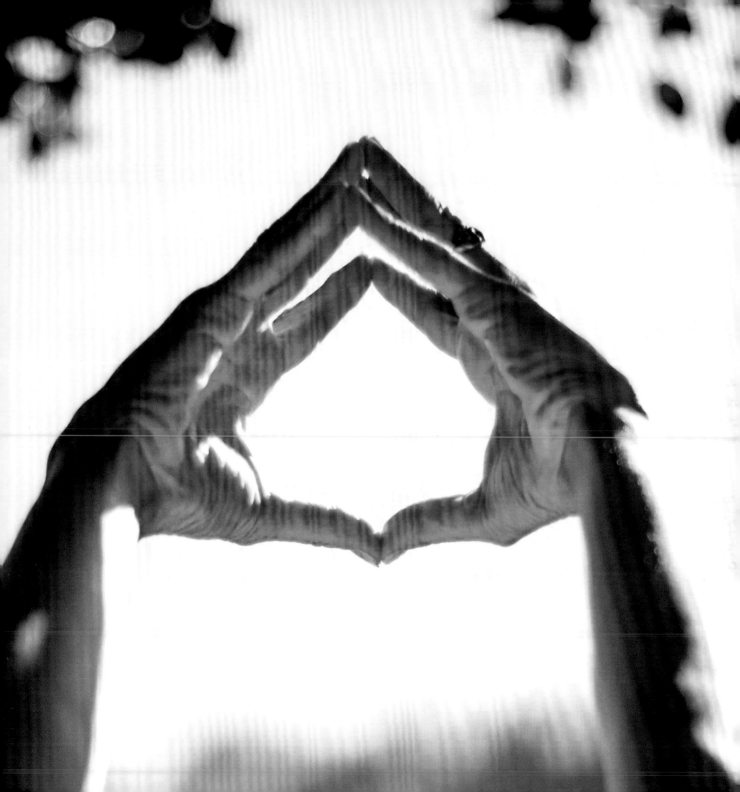

CHAPTER SEVEN
THE SEQUENCES

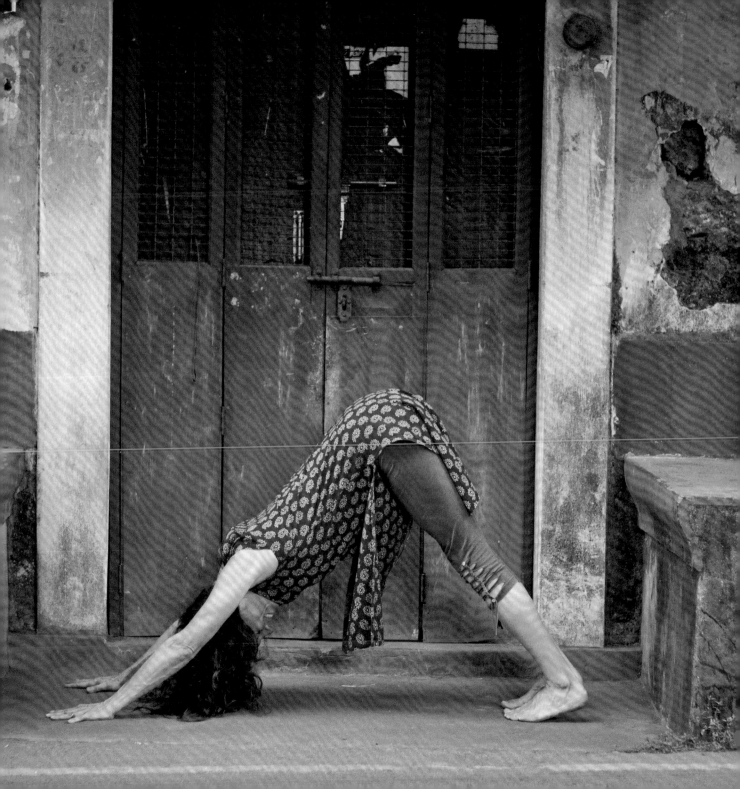

| Choosing your sequence

Phew! You made it! You're ready to find the practice that's right for you. A few more steps and you're there.

Step 1

If you haven't done so yet, take the Ayurvedic dosha questionnaire, on the following spread, to find your current condition (vikruti).

Add up the number of points in the two sections:

1. Body imbalance 2. Mind

The highest number is the dominant dosha. So for example, if you score 18 points for Pitta, 12 for Vata and 8 for Kapha, your vikruti is Pitta/Vata which means you would start with the Pitta sequence.

Step 2

Go to the practice chart and find your dominant dosha and the associated sequence, breathing and meditation practices, and recommended daily routine. Explore that practice for at least 7 to 14 days.

Step 3

If a posture is too challenging, check out the variation on the same page or head to the modification section at the back of the book. You can also skip it. Some postures are designed to prepare you for the more challenging ones. Start with the ones you feel you can do and build slowly. You may not believe it now, but even one week of daily practice will make a difference. All you have to do is show up. Your body will take care of the rest.

| What is your dosha?

| HOW TO USE THIS QUESTIONNAIRE

As you go through the descriptions for each dosha, place a check mark beside the one that best describes you. Make sure your answers are based on your current condition. If you are presenting symptoms from two or more of the doshas score a half-point for each.

Next, add up the score for the body and the mind seperately. Then add the body and mind together for your final score. If you have an equal score for two of the doshas then go back to the separate scores for body and mind and look at which one is more dominant.

For example, if your body is presenting with a high number of Pitta symptoms, choose the Pitta sequence to calm and soothe the fire. If your mind is presenting with more Vata symptoms, choose the Vata sequence to ground and restore the nervous system. You can repeat the questionnaire as your current condition changes.

BODY	✔	VATA	✔	PITTA	✔	KAPHA
Weight	○	usually thin ribs visible can vary	○	medium	○	larger hard to lose weight
Skin	○	dry rough cool thin	○	oily smooth warm moles present rosy	○	thick cool oily pale
Hair	○	thin dry kinky	○	oily reddish balding grey	○	thick luxurious oily wavy
Eyes	○	smaller blinking nervous scanty lashes	○	intense piercing light-sensitive the white part is often reddish or yellow	○	larger beautiful thick lashes calm
Teeth	○	irregular- spaces or too many teeth protruding crooked	○	moderate gums bleed easily	○	nicely formed white and healthy gums receding
Joints	○	crack easily stiff	○	moderate-sized loose	○	larger and firm
Circulation	○	variable to poor	○	good strong	○	moderate
Appetite	○	variable irregular	○	strong to excessive	○	steady but slower
Stool	○	irregular gas constipated hard	○	regular movement soft loose burns	○	large well-formed
Thirst	○	scanty irregular	○	strong excessive	○	moderate
BODY TOTAL						

MIND	✔	VATA	✔	PITTA	✔	KAPHA
Emotions		enthusiastic tends to worry		intense courageous quick to anger fear		calm slow to anger can be possessive and over-attached
Temperament		changeable variable		motivated driven competitive impatient		easy going
Speech		fast frequent		good orators can be sharp or argumentative		slower or more silent
Mind		very quick curious adaptable loses interest quickly restless		penetrating critical sharp intellect		slower lethargic
Faith		variable erratic		determined strong possibly fanatical		steady, slow to change
Memory		quick but absent minded		clear sharp learns and forgets easily		slow and steady
Sleep		disturbed poor light		medium		heavy to excess
MIND TOTAL						
BODY/MIND TOTAL						

PRACTICE CHART

VIKRUTI/CURRENT CONDITION	ASANA SEQUENCE	BREATHING
Vata/Pitta	Vata balancing	Full complete breath
Pitta/Vata	Pitta balancing	Ocean breath
Vata/Kapha	Vata balancing	Alternate nostril breath
Vata	Vata balancing	Full complete breath
Pitta	Pitta balancing	Alternate nostril breath
Kapha	Kapha balancing	Ocean breath
Kapha/Pitta	Kapha balancing	Full complete breath
Kapha/Vata	Kapha balancing	Alternate nostril breath
Pitta/Kapha	Pitta balancing	Alternate nostril breath
Vata/Pitta/Kapha	Vata balancing	Full complete breath

MEDITATION	BEST TIME OF DAY FOR PRACTICE	DAILY ROUTINE
Sunrise	Between 6am and 10am	Sesame oil on feet and head
Satyam	Between 6am and 10am	Yoga nidra (20 min)
Soham	Before 6am	Walk in the early morning or after dinner
Sunrise	Between 6am and 10am, or 6pm and 10pm	Sesame oil on feet and head
Soham	Between 6am and 10am	Yoga nidra (20 min)
Satyam	Before 6am or between 2pm and 6pm	Walk in the early morning or after dinner
Sunrise	Before 6am or between 2pm and 6pm	Walk in the early morning or after dinner
Soham	Before 6am	Walk in the early morning or after dinner
Satyam	Before 6am or between 2pm and 6pm	Yoga nidra (20 min)
Sunrise	Between 6am and 10am, or 6pm and 10pm	Sesame oil on feet and head

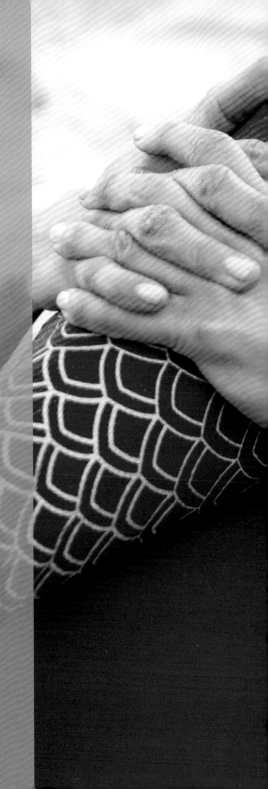

THINK OF THE VATA CONSTITUTION AS A BUTTERFLY: LIGHT, FREE, DELICATE, SENSITIVE AND INCREDIBLY BEAUTIFUL

INTENTION

MAY I BE GROUNDED, NURTURED AND RESTORED

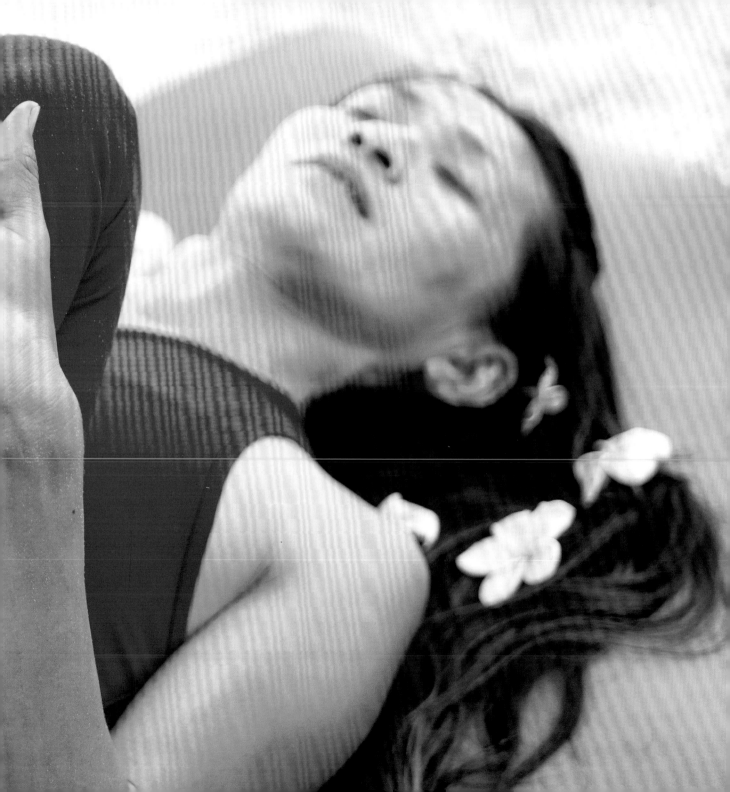

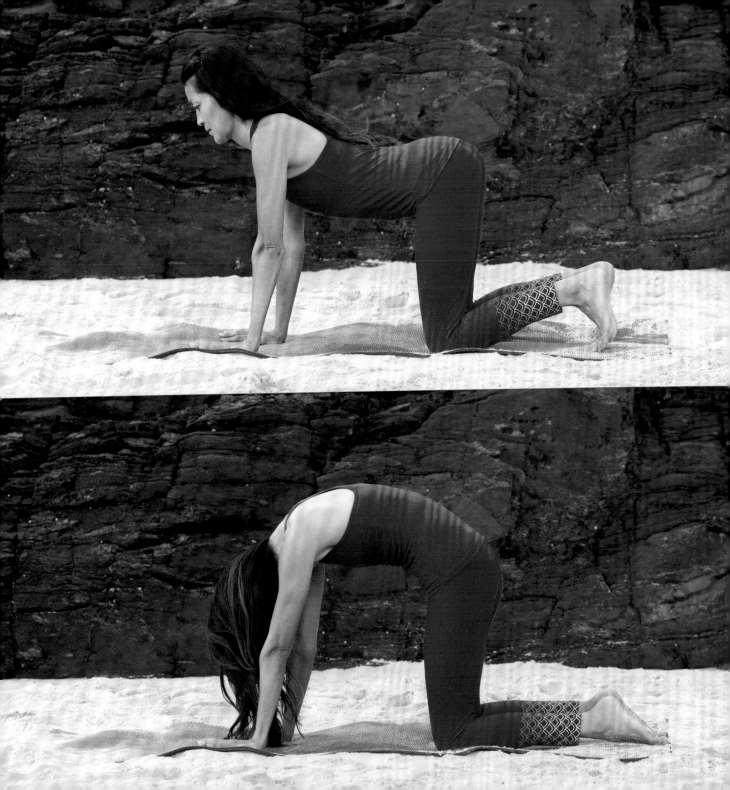

| MOVING CAT POSE

WARM-UP
FOCUS
RELEASE
LUBRICATE

Come onto your hands and knees.

Place your hands underneath your shoulders and your knees underneath your hips.

Tuck the toes under inhale and expand your upper chest forward keeping the lower abdominals engaged and the lower spine in neutral.

Exhale relax the tops of the feet to the ground, round through the lower spine and completely relax the head.

Repeat the movement inhaling opening the chest and exhaling rounding the lower spine.

Feel the breath and movement working together.

Benefits

Moving Cat posture is the perfect way to warm up the spine. Because it involves a backbend and a forward bend, moving the spine through extension and flexion.

Focusing on the breath inspires focus

Releases any tightness behind the upper back, shoulders and lower back

The perfect way to learn how to coordinate breath and movement.

Variations

If you have wrist issues practice on your forearms.

If you have knee pain, place a blanket under your knees.

| CHILD POSE

Benefits

Child pose is a neutral position for your spine.

Your head is below your heart, which lowers your blood pressure.

It massages the internal organs.

It's nourishing for the kidneys and adrenals, because the breath is directed towards the back of the body.

A great resting posture.

Variations

Place a block under your forehead, if your head does not easily touch the floor.

Place a bolster or rolled up blanket behind your knees to create more space, if you're tight in the thighs.

Reach the arms out in front of you placing your palms shoulder-width apart to make the pose more active.

Start on your hands and knees.

Exhaling, send your buttocks back to your heels.

Rest your chest to your thighs, forehead on the ground and have your hands alongside your body.

Breathe here, feeling the belly pressed against the thighs and the skin on the back of the body stretching.

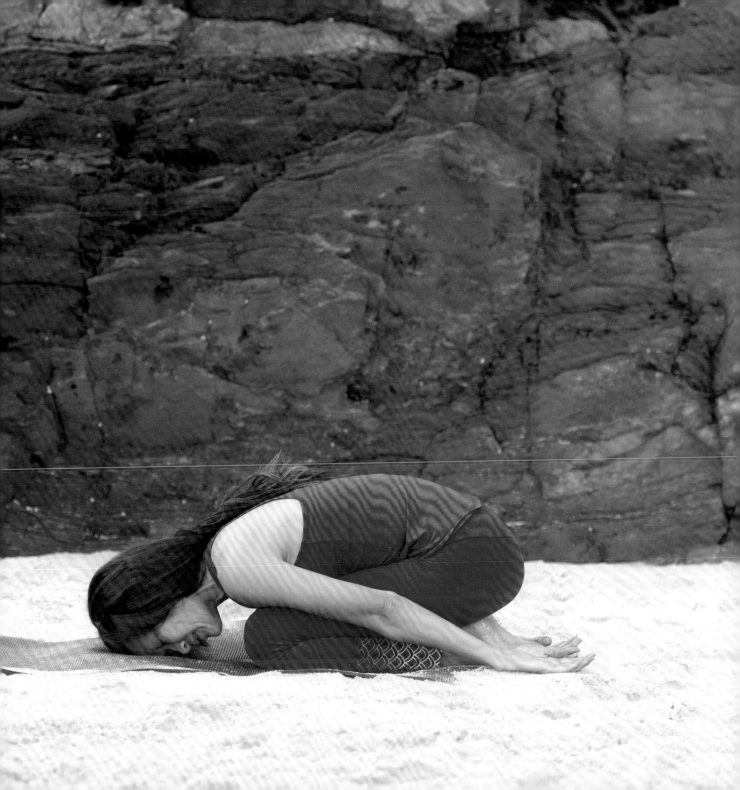

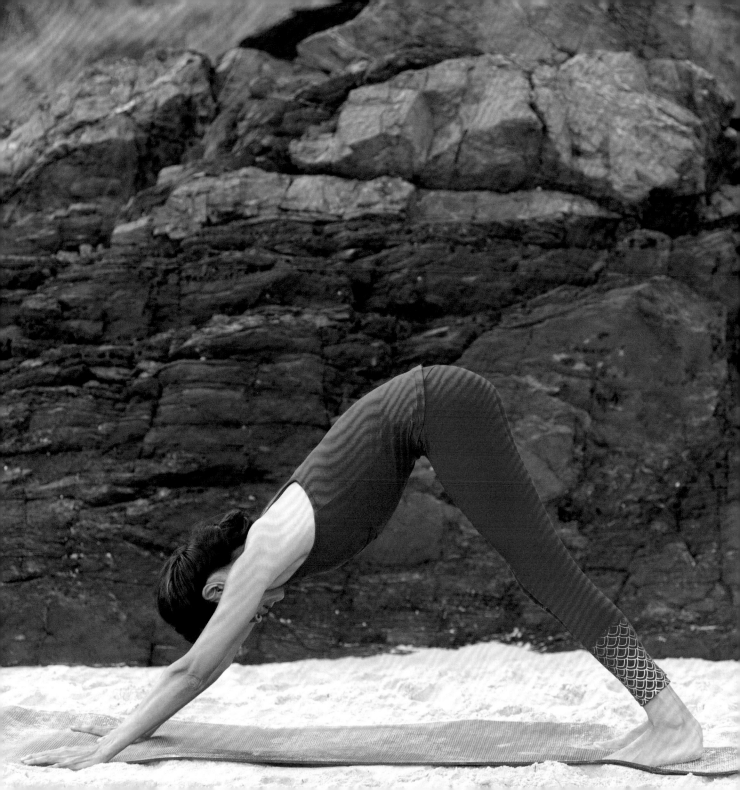

| DOWN DOG POSE

Start in Child pose.

Reach your arms out in front of you spreading your fingers wide, the crease line of your wrist lined up with the end of your mat.

Tuck your toes under and, as you exhale, lift your buttocks towards the sky. If you're tight in the hamstrings, bend your knees.

If your spine is rounding and you feel too much weight in your arms, bend your knees more.

It should feel like you're pushing your hands away from the ground, extending your sitting bones (the point where your buttocks meet your leg) to the sky.

Feel the length in your spine and the space in between each vertebra.

On your next exhalation, come down and rest in Child pose.

Benefits

Down Dog stretches and lengthens the spine.

The head is lower than the heart so the nervous system relaxes.

It opens the hamstrings.

Releases the shoulders.

Strengthens the wrists and forearms.

It brings awareness to your breath and facilitates better breathing.

It challenges you to go beyond limitations; as you hold the pose and the arms get tired, staying there that little bit longer pushes you to the edge of your perceived boundaries.

Variations

Bend your knees if your hamstrings are tight or you feel pulling in your lower back.

| FULL FORWARD FOLD

CALM
INVERT
REST
REVIVE

Start in Down Dog.

Walk your feet to your hands.

Bend your knees so that your belly rests on your thighs.

Fold your arms as they hang below your head, placing the thumbs in the elbow crease and wrapping the remaining four fingers around the outside of the elbows.

Breathe deeply keeping the connection between the belly and the thighs.

Feel the skin on the back of your body stretching and the breath reaching into the kidney area.

After a few rounds of breath, release your arms so they dangle towards the ground.

On your next inhalation, keep the knees bent and slowly roll up, stacking one vertebra on top of the other. Feel like a fern uncurling.

Let your head be the last thing to come up.

Exhale in the standing position.

Benefits

Full Forward Fold lowers blood pressure and calms the mind because the head is below the heart.

It releases and stretches the hamstring muscles.

Massages the internal organs.

Releases the shoulders.

A great resting position.

Variations

Bend the knees more, if your belly doesn't easily reach your thighs.

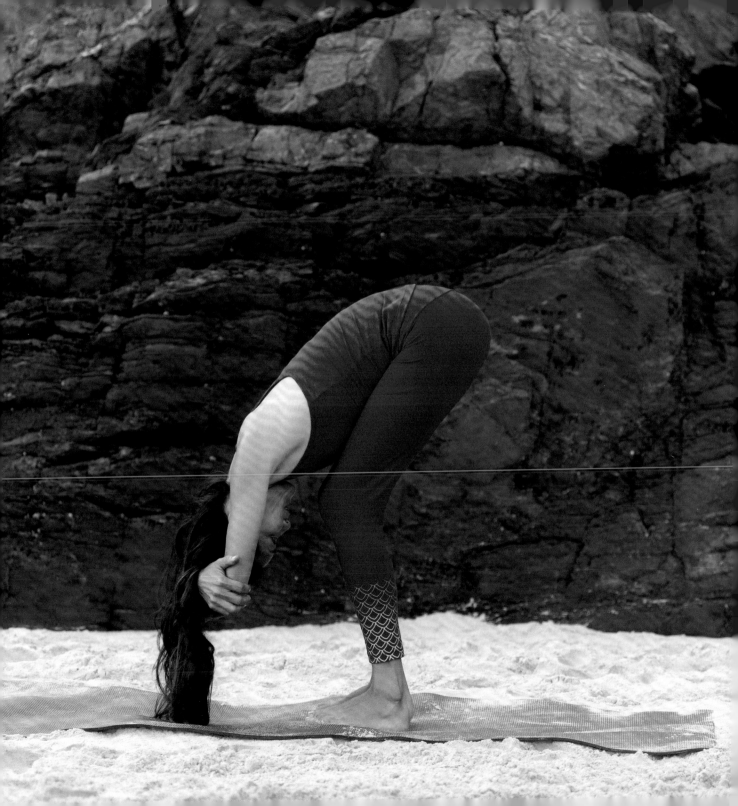

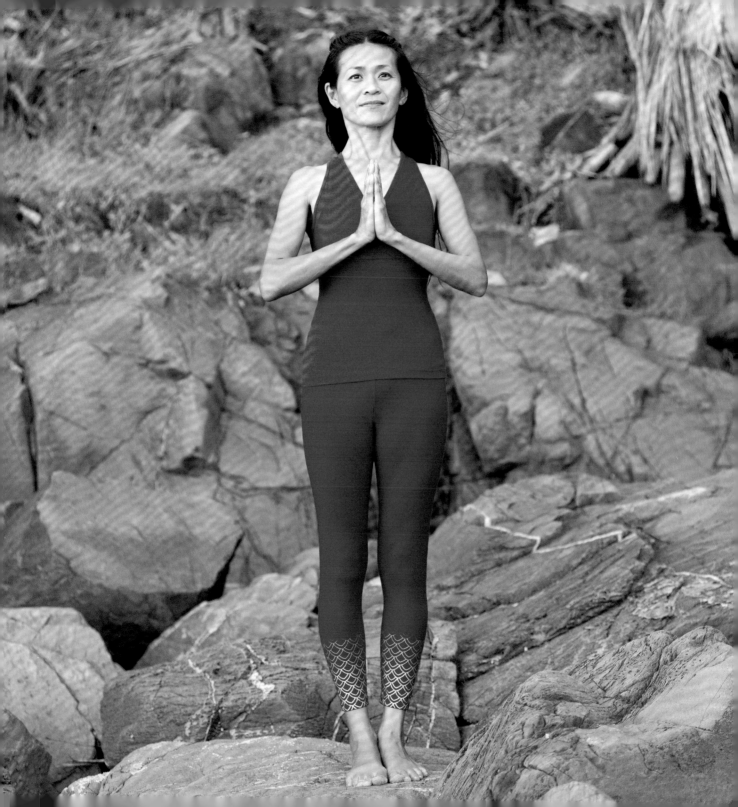

| MOUNTAIN POSE

Stand with the big toes touching and the heels slightly apart.

Feel the weight balanced between the four corners of the foot: the outer heel, little toe mound, big toe mound and inner heel.

Engage the thighs keeping the knees soft.

Feel your tailbone lengthening.

Create space between the top of your hipbones and the base of your ribcage.

Open the chest, relax the shoulders and keep the chin level.

Bring the hands into prayer position.

Benefits

Mountain pose is one of the safest positions for the spine.

The weight is balanced between both feet which supports the spine in maintaining its natural curves.

This means there is no significant strain in any part of the body.

This pose supports the body in bearing weight.

It facilitates easy and open breathing.

A calming posture.

Perfect resting pose between the standing postures.

Variations

Relax the arms alongside the body, slightly roll the upper arms out and the forearms in.

Interlace the fingers in front of the chest and raise the arms up over the head.

| WARRIOR 2 POSE

Stand at the top of your mat in Mountain pose, big toes touching, heels slightly apart.

Take a big step back with your left leg and face towards the left side of your mat.

Line up your right heel with the middle arch of your left foot.

Bend your front knee placing your hands on your hips.

Make sure your front knee is over your ankle in a stacked position.

Look down and make sure you can still see all five toes and the top half of your front foot. (If you can't, you've bent your knee too much.)

Check to make sure your front knee isn't rolling in or out.

Turn in your back hip and foot to keep the front knee tracking over the ankle.

Raise your arms to shoulder height and gaze over your right middle finger.

Take 5 deep breaths in the posture.

On your next exhalation, straighten the front leg turn both feet to the center.

Repeat on the other side.

Benefits

Warrior 2 posture builds strength and stamina.

It strengthens the knee joint and powers up the front thigh.

It facilitates deep breathing in the chest.

Strengthens the upper body.

Opens the hip flexor of the back leg.

Variations

Line up the front heel with the back heel if your hips are tight.

Decrease the bend in the front knee if the posture feels too strong or there is strain in your knee joint.

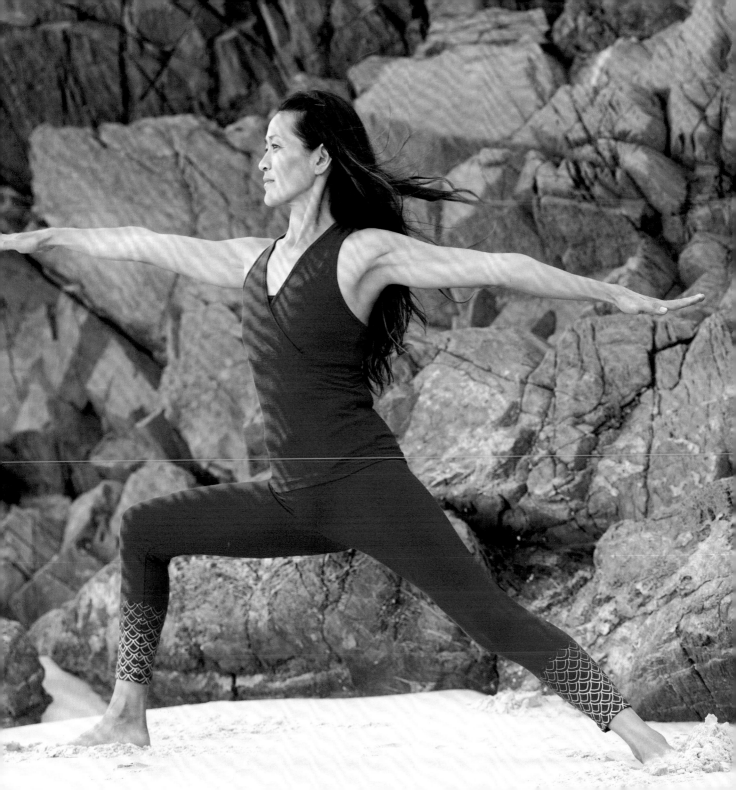

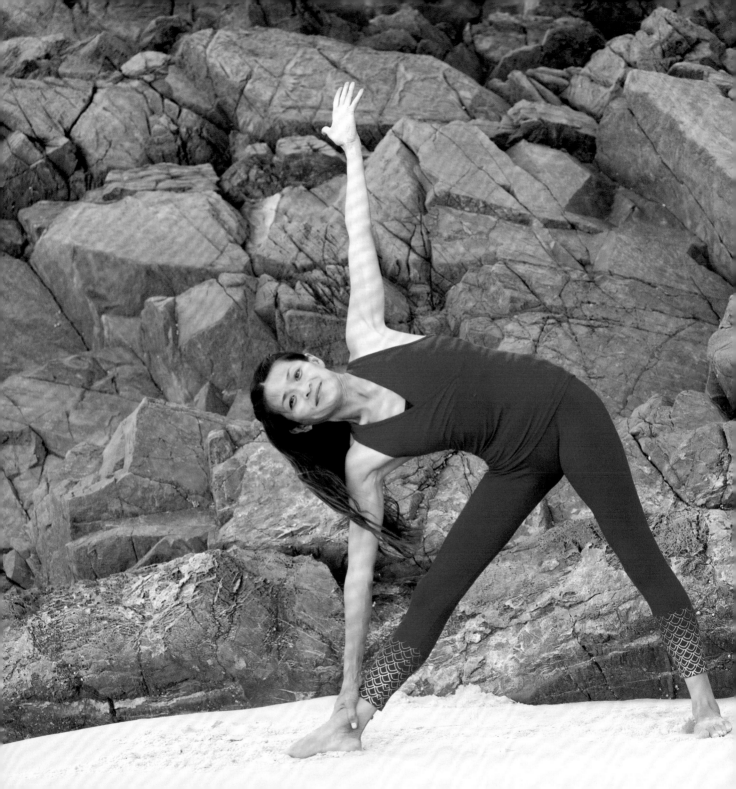

| TRIANGLE POSE

Stand at the top of your mat in Mountain pose, big toes touching, heels slightly apart.

Take a medium step back with your left leg and face towards the left side of your mat.

Line up your right heel with the middle arch of your left foot.

Place your hands on your hips.

Turn your hips slightly so that you face towards your front leg.

Raise the arms to shoulder height and shift the left hip back while deepening the front hip crease.

Feel the hip of the front leg drawing back while the hip of the back leg rolls down to face the floor. (This action helps to release the lower back and increases the length in the underneath side of the torso.)

As the spine lengthens over the front thigh, reach the bottom hand on to the ankle and raise the top arm, lining up the wrist with the shoulder.

Inhale and open the chest more, gazing straight ahead.

Take 5 deep breaths in the posture.

On your next exhalation, ground down into your front foot, inhale and bring the torso upright. Turn both feet to the center.

Repeat on the other side.

STRETCH
OPEN
TONE
EXTEND

Benefits

Triangle pose increases the stretch on the front inner thigh and opens the hamstrings.

It opens the hips.

Increases breath capacity.

Tones the muscles around the kidneys.

Stretches the muscles responsible for side bending.

Variations

Bend the front knee slightly, if there is strain in the front knee or inner thigh.

Place your hand on your shin, if it doesn't easily reach your ankle.

| TRIANGLE FORWARD BEND

Stand at the top of your mat in Mountain pose, big toes touching, heels slightly apart.

Take a medium step back with your left leg keeping both hips facing the front of the mat.

Place your hands on your hips, inhale and lift your chest towards the sky.

As you exhale, fold forward at the hip crease, extending the spine until your belly and your front thigh meet.

Rest your hands on either side of your front foot.

Take 5 to 10 deep breaths here.

Take your hands back to your hips.

Ground down into your feet.

Inhaling, bring the torso back upright.

Step the left foot to the top of the mat and repeat on the other side.

Benefits

Triangle Forward Bend creates a deep stretch in the front hamstring.

The connection between the front thigh and the belly massages the internal organs.

A great calming posture.

Variation

Place the hands on blocks underneath the shoulders and bend the front knee slightly if the front hamstring is tight.

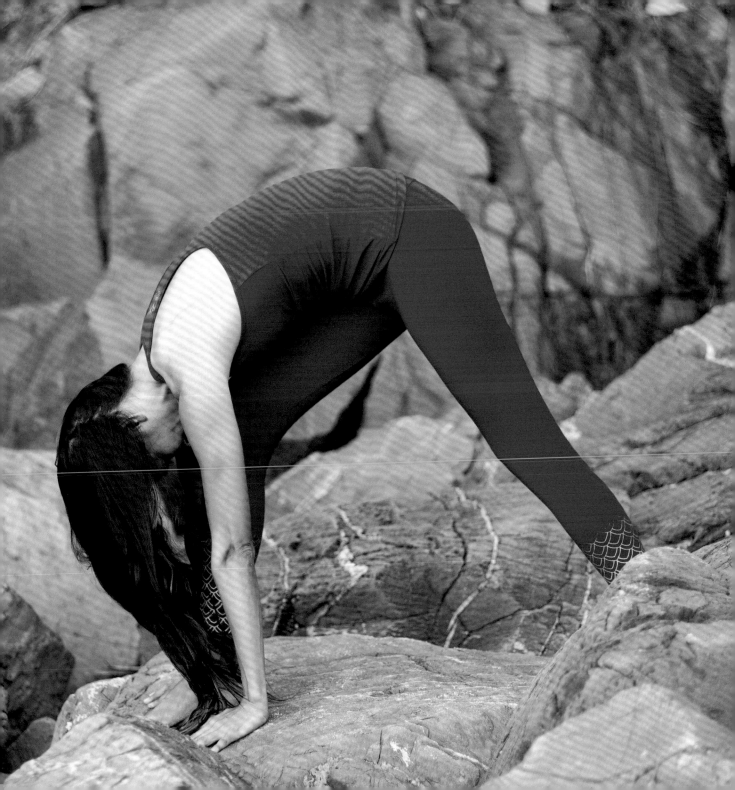

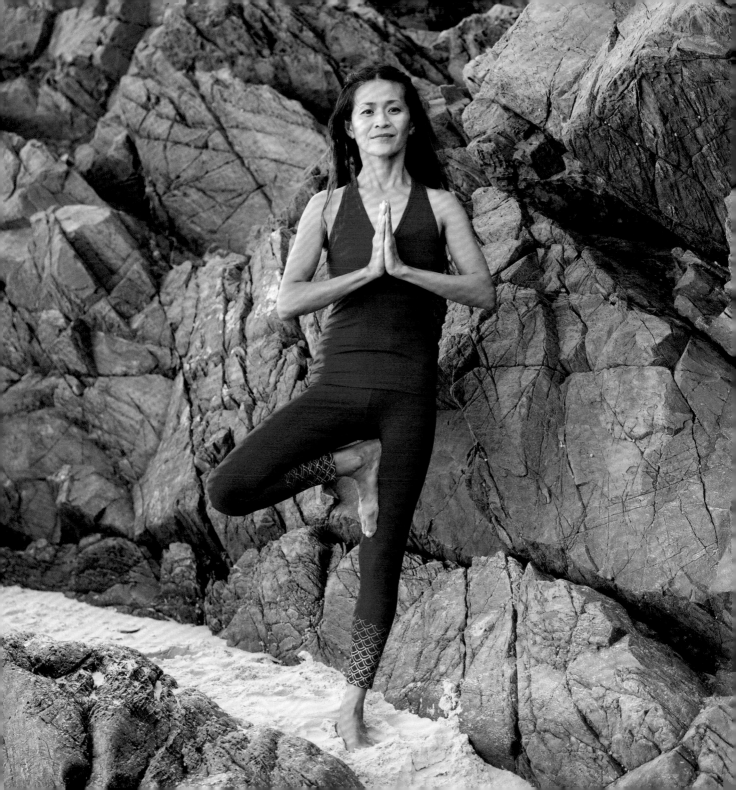

| TREE POSE

STRENGTH
BROADEN
SOOTHE
BALANCE

Stand at the top of your mat in Mountain pose, big toes touching, heels slightly apart.

Shift the weight to the right leg and gently place the left heel on the right ankle pressing the ball of the left foot into the floor.

Next, place the left foot along the inside of the right shin.

If you feel balanced, grip the left ankle with your left hand and place the left foot against the right inner thigh where the groin and top thigh meet.

Your hips are level and face the top of the mat while your knee comes forward slightly.

Place your hands in prayer position at your heart, open your chest, relax your shoulders.

Breathe deeply gazing at a point either straight ahead or slightly down in front of you.

Release the foot and come back to Mountain pose.

Repeat on the other side.

Benefits

Tree pose strengthens the ankle and foot.

It opens the hip of the bent leg.

Develops balance.

It's soothing for the nervous system.

A calming and cooling posture.

Variations

Place the left heel on the right ankle, pressing the ball of the foot into the floor.

Take the arms over head pressing palms together.

| SPHINX POSE

OPEN
STIMULATE
BREATHE
FREEDOM

Lie on your belly, forehead pressing into the ground, arms relaxed alongside the body with your thighs, knees and toes all facing down.

Come up onto your forearms so that the elbows are slightly forward of the shoulders and wider than shoulder-width.

Feel your ribcage lifting off the ground while the belly button still touches the ground.

Open through the front of the chest, lengthening and extending the spine.

Activate the inner thighs and lift them towards the sky while relaxing the buttocks.

Keep the neck in line with the spine and your gaze out in front.

Breathe deeply into the chest and hold for 5 to 10 breaths.

Benefits

Sphinx pose strengthens your legs, back, arms and shoulders.

It stretches the front of the body and opens the psoas muscle (the muscle connecting the upper half of the body to the lower half).

It supports the body in taking deep chest breaths.

Improves digestion.

Tones the kidneys and adrenals.

A stimulating and awakening posture.

Variations

Walk the hands further away from the chest, lift the elbows and straighten the arms, if there is any discomfort in the lower back.

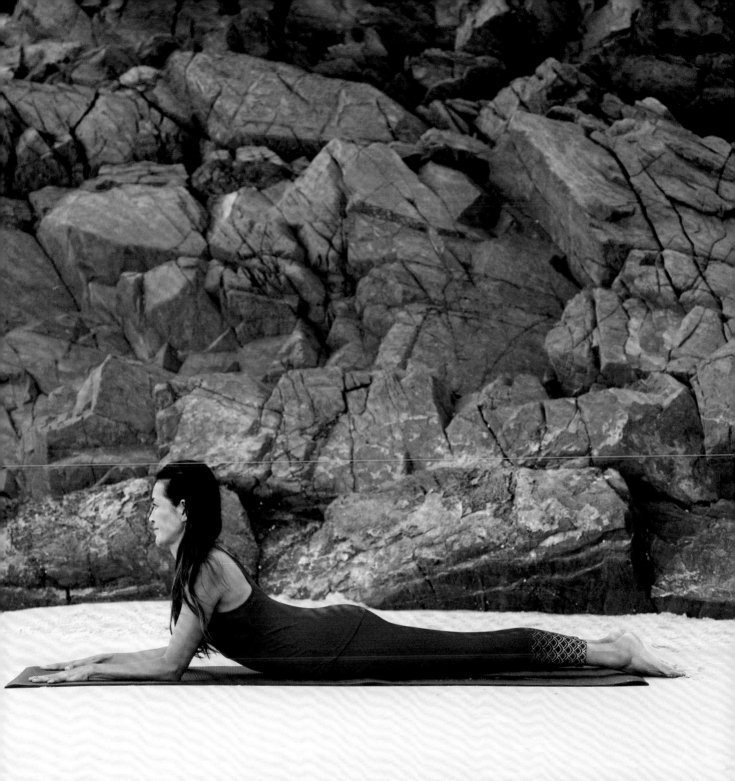

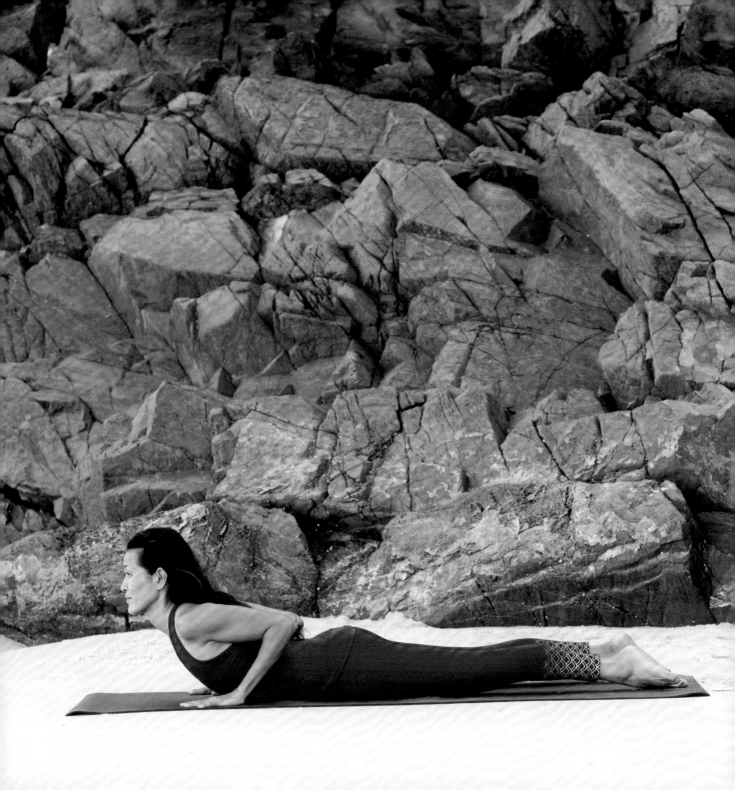

| BABY COBRA POSE

TONE
MASSAGE
ENGAGE
WIDEN

Lie on your belly, forehead pressing into the ground, arms relaxed alongside the body with your thighs, knees and toes all facing down.

Place the hands beside your chest and have the thumbs in line with the center of your chest at the nipple line, elbows tucked close into the body and pointing backwards.

Activate the abdominals and the pelvic floor and lengthen the lower back.

Activate the inner thighs and lift them towards the sky while relaxing the buttocks.

Lift the front of the chest, keeping the bottom of your ribs, entire abdomen and pubic bone on the ground.

Keep your neck in line with your spine.

Gaze forwards.

Take 5 to 10 breaths here.

Come down, turn your head to one side, rest on your cheek and relax.

Benefits

Baby Cobra works the muscles on either side of the spine, toning the kidneys and adrenals.

It massages the internal organs.

Engages the breath in your upper chest.

Releases the lower back, while working the hamstrings.

An energizing and stimulating pose.

Variations

Tuck the toes under and lift the knees to activate the quadriceps (front thigh muscles).

Lift the feet and hands off the floor.

Move on the breath, inhaling lifting into the pose, exhaling relaxing back down.

| CHILD POSE VARIATION

Come to sit upright on your heels with your knees together.

Keep the big toes touching as you take your knees wide apart.

Gently walk your hands forward.

Extend your spine while drawing the shoulder blades onto your back.

Hands are shoulder-width apart.

Rest your forehead on the floor. (If it's uncomfortable, turn your cheek to one side.)

Stay here for a few minutes.

Relaxing Visualization

Become aware of your breath.

Feel the breath filling the belly, ribs and upper chest.

Become aware of your heartbeat.

Visualize a rose in your right hand.

Twirl the stem of the rose between your forefinger and thumb.

As you twirl the rose, imagine you are close enough to see the colored petals of the rose laced in delicate dew drops, and imagine its fragrance is rich and sweet.

Become so focused on the rose that you almost feel yourself becoming the rose.

Once again, become aware of your heartbeat.

Come back to your breath, feeling it fill your belly, ribs and upper chest.

Slowly come up and be ready for the next pose.

🔊 https://soundcloud.com/the-flying-yogini/rose-meditation

STRETCH RESTORE REST REPLENISH

Benefits

This calming, restorative pose lowers blood pressure.

It rejuvenates your spine and releases your lower back.

It slows the breath down so that the nervous system takes deep rest.

It can be practiced whenever you need to slow down your breath.

A gentle hip-opener and thigh stretch.

Variations

Place a bolster or rolled up blanket behind the knees, if you are tight in the thighs.

Place your forehead on a block, if you find it hard to lengthen your spine.

Bring your knees closer together, if you are tight in your hips.

Take your knees wider apart for a deeper stretch.

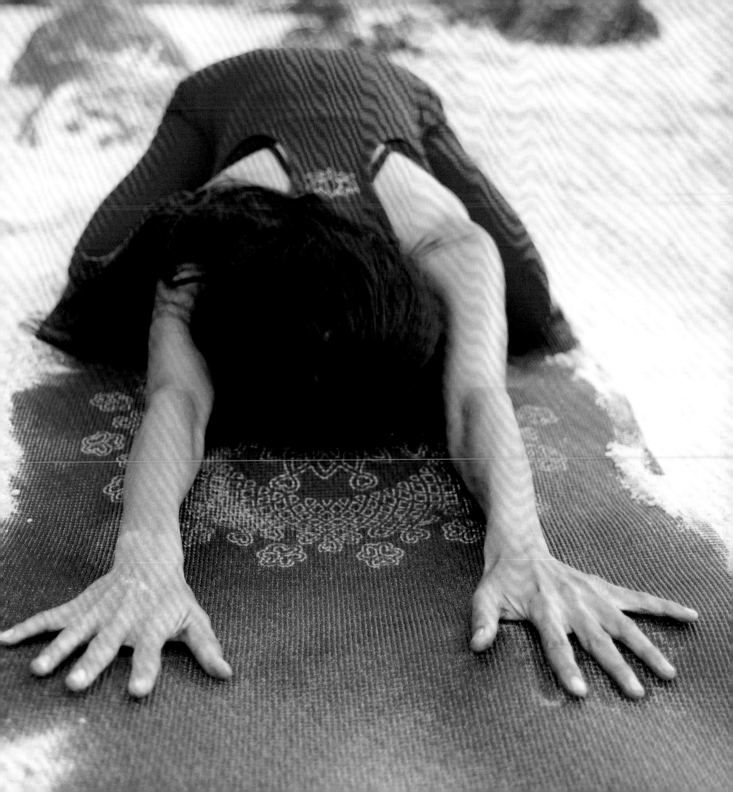

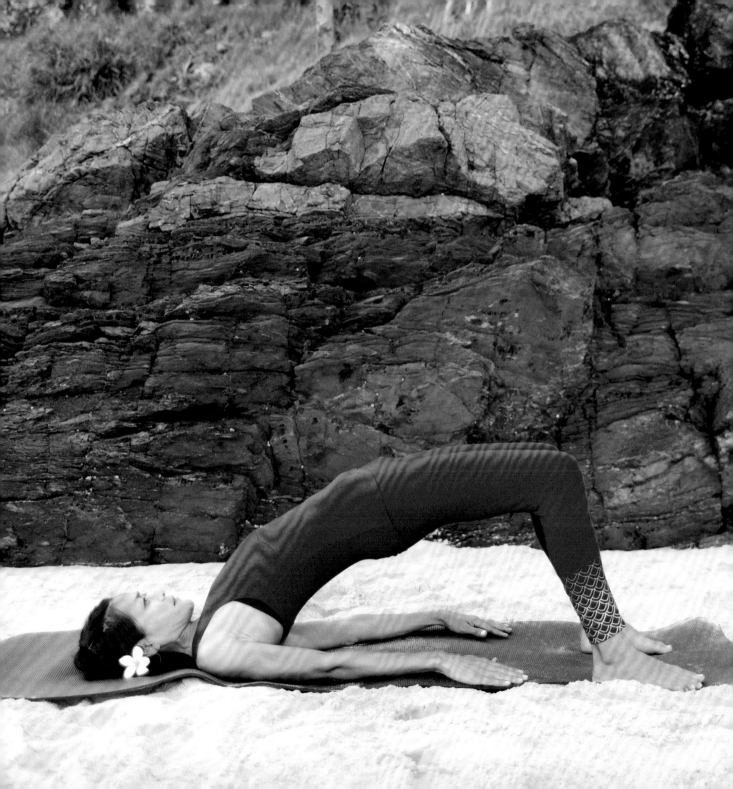

| BRIDGE POSE

EXPAND
ENERGIZE
BREATHE
SUPPORT

Lie on your back with your knees bent and feet flat on the ground.

Have your feet slightly in front of your knees and a little wider than hip-width apart.

Exhale and tuck your tailbone under slightly.

Inhaling, lift your pelvis towards the sky.

Gently roll in your thighs, toes slightly turned in and feel your tailbone lengthening.

The lower back should feel free and open, with the buttocks soft.

Lift your chest towards your chin, then draw the chin a little bit away from the chest to create a curve in the back of your neck.

Breathe here watching your belly rise and fall.

Once you are in the pose, do not move your head or neck.

Hold for 5 to 10 breaths, then slowly come down rolling inch by inch through each vertebra.

Rest with the knees together and the feet wide at the outer edges of the mat.

Benefits

Bridge pose stretches the tops of your thighs.

It releases the lower back.

It facilitates deep breathing because there is no pressure on the diaphragm.

It expands the chest area.

It's energizing for the spine.

It helps balance your metabolism due to the stimulation of the thyroid gland (in the throat).

Variations

Rest your lower back on a block if this pose strains the knees, hurts the lower back or you have neck issues.

| WIND EXPELLER POSE

STRETCH
MASSAGE
RELAX
CLEAR

Lie on your back with the legs extended and parallel to each other.

Feel your length from the crown of your head to your tailbone.

Bend the right knee and interlace the fingers over the shin.

Gently draw the thigh towards your chest.

Keep your heel in line with your knee.

Flex evenly through both feet, activating the legs.

Draw the tailbone down to the floor, feeling the lower back lengthening along the floor.

As you breathe in and out, feel the right side of your belly receiving a deep massage.

Hold here for 5 to 10 breaths.

Release the leg and repeat on the other side.

Benefits

Wind Expeller stretches the psoas muscle on the extended leg side and activates the psoas muscle on the bent leg side.

It provides a massage for the ascending colon on the right side and descending colon on the left side.

It facilitates relaxation and letting go.

Releases wind and balances the air element in the body.

Wonderful to do before bed or even lying in bed.

Variations

Bend the extended leg at the knee and rest the foot flat on the ground, if there are any lower back issues.

Loop a strap around the front of the shin and hold onto either end, if you can't comfortably hold your thigh.

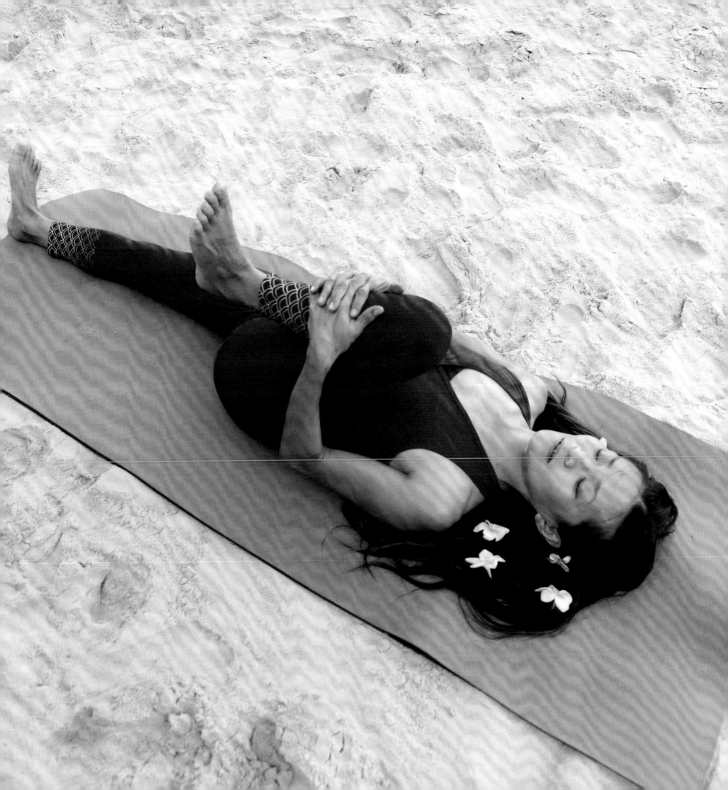

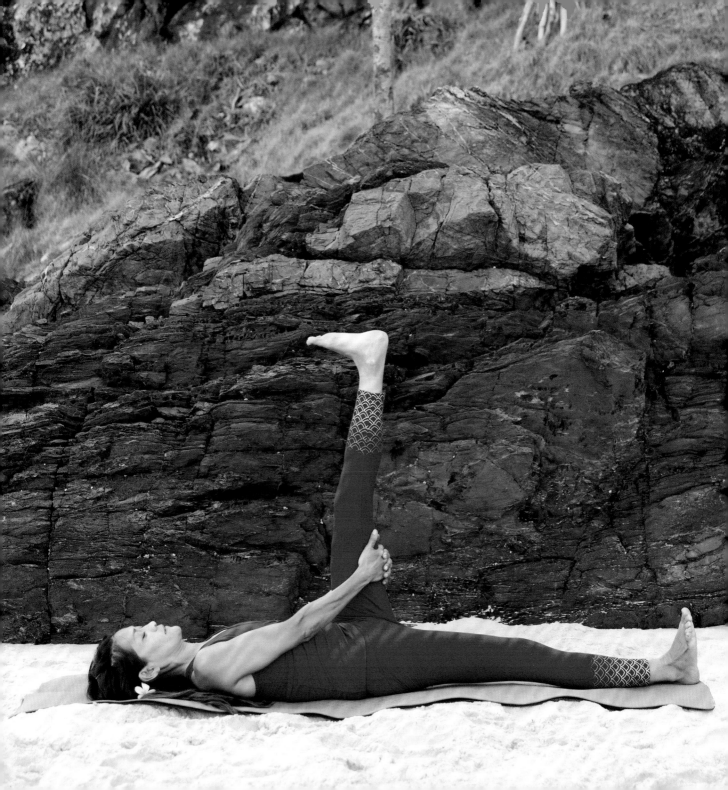

| RESTING EXTENDED LEG POSE

Lie on your back with the legs extended and parallel to each other.

Feel length from the crown of your head to your tailbone.

Bend the right knee and interlace the fingers behind the thigh.

Extend the foot to the sky keeping the leg straight and the thigh muscle engaged.

Press the back of your thigh into your hands and your hands into your thigh creating a feeling of resistance. (This will co-activate the muscles around the thigh bone and increase the effectiveness of the stretch.)

Make sure the leg along the ground is straight with the knee facing towards the sky.

Flex both feet.

Breathe deeply into the chest.

Hold here for 5 to 10 breaths.

Release the leg and repeat on the other side.

Benefits

Resting Extended Leg pose is one of the safest and most effective ways to open the hamstrings as there is no pressure on the lower back.

It releases tension in the lower back and hamstring muscles.

Relaxes the nervous system.

When you actively press your thigh into your hands and your hands into your thigh, you tone the muscles of the upper arms and upper chest.

Variation

Bend the knee of the raised leg, if there is any tension in the hamstrings.

| COBBLER POSE

Benefits

Cobbler pose is a deep inner thigh stretch.

It increases circulation to your pelvis.

It works the abdominals to support the spine in the upright position.

Works the buttock muscles.

Pressing the soles of the feet together firmly strengthens the knees.

It supports your reproductive and hormonal system.

A calming and grounding posture.

Come to sit on your sitting bones.

Bend both knees and place the soles of the feet together a comfortable distance away from the groin. (If you've made a diamond shape with the legs, the feet are too far away from the groin.)

Grasp the ankles with your hands.

Sit tall and gently squeeze the buttocks towards each other which will enable the thighs to move closer towards the ground.

Breathe deeply into the chest.

Hold here for 10 to 15 breaths.

Feel tension melting away and just be content with holding the posture as it is.

Variations

If the thighs are tight, bring the feet further away from the groin into a diamond shape.

To increase the stretch, bring the feet as close to the groin as possible.

If the knees are way above the hips, sit on a block or bolster.

If the back is rounding, sit against a wall.

This pose can be practiced lying down.

Lie on your back, bend the knees and bring the soles of the feet together.

Close your eyes and relax.
(This posture is in the Pitta sequence p.236)

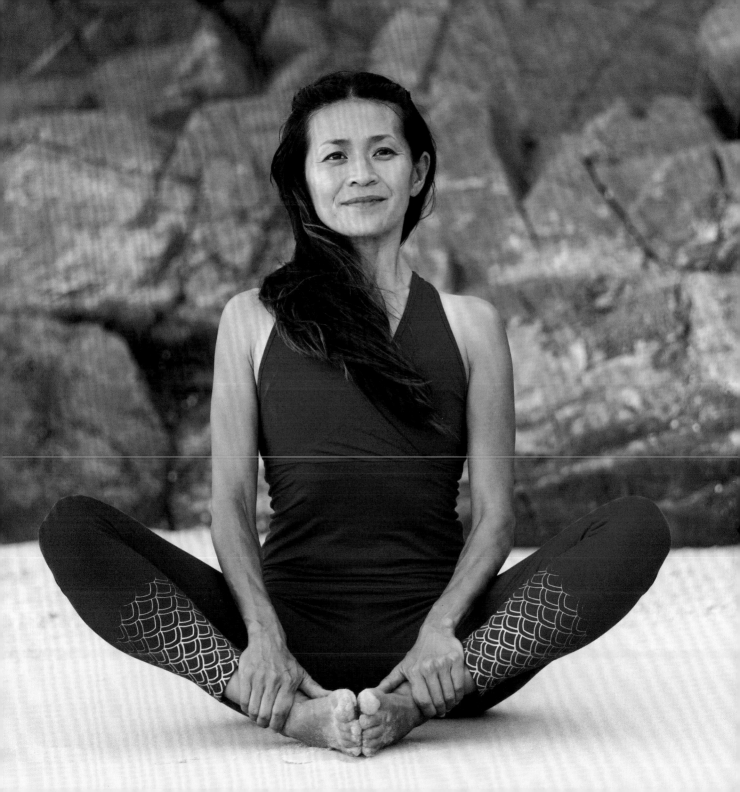

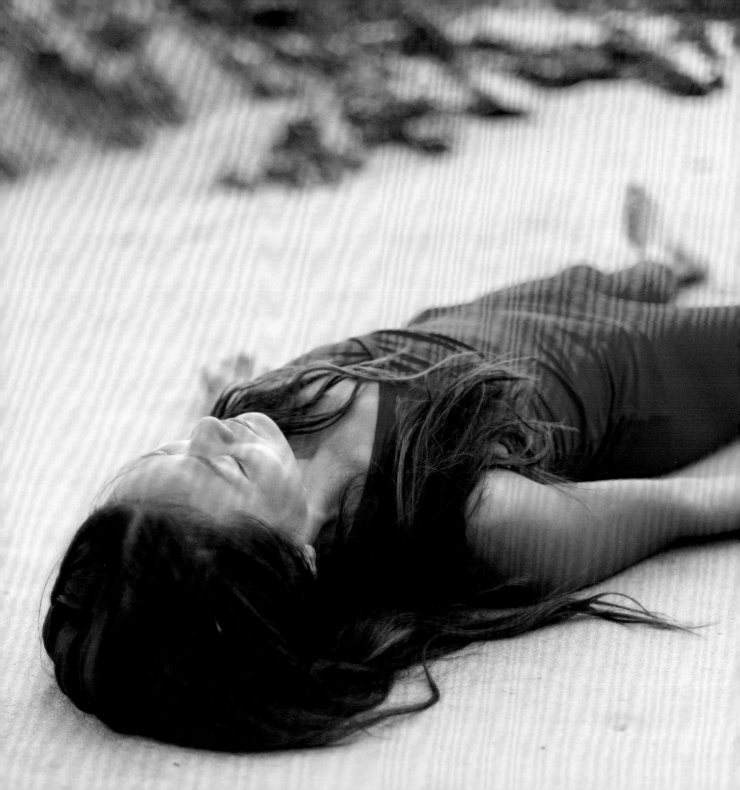

| CORPSE POSE

NOURISH
RELAX
RELEASE
REPLENISH

Lie on your back.

Have your arms and legs slightly away from the body, palms facing upwards, feet relaxed and open.

Turn the head gently from side to side until it rests in the center.

If your chin juts up towards the sky, place a blanket underneath your head.

Relax completely.

Don't worry about the breath or what the body is doing.

Feel how effortless it is to lie here.

Stay here for at least 5 minutes.

When you are ready, roll to one side and come up.

Benefits

This is the most important posture in the sequence. Missing this posture is like making a meal and then deciding not to eat it.

All the nourishing and healing benefits of the practice are integrated in this posture.

The relaxed part of the nervous system is engaged.

The body releases and relaxes at a cellular level.

The glandular system is replenished.

The alpha and theta brainwaves are dominant and the mind relaxes.

Variations

Place a bolster under your knees, if there is pressure in your lower back.

Place an inch-thick folded blanket under the head, if there is any tension in the neck.

Place an eye pillow over your eyes if you have an active mind.

A PITTA TYPE IS COMFORTABLE IN A LEADERSHIP ROLE. THEY ARE CHARISMATIC, RADIANT AND ADMIRED BY THEIR PEERS.

INTENTION

MAY I FEEL SOOTHED, CALM AND SURRENDERED

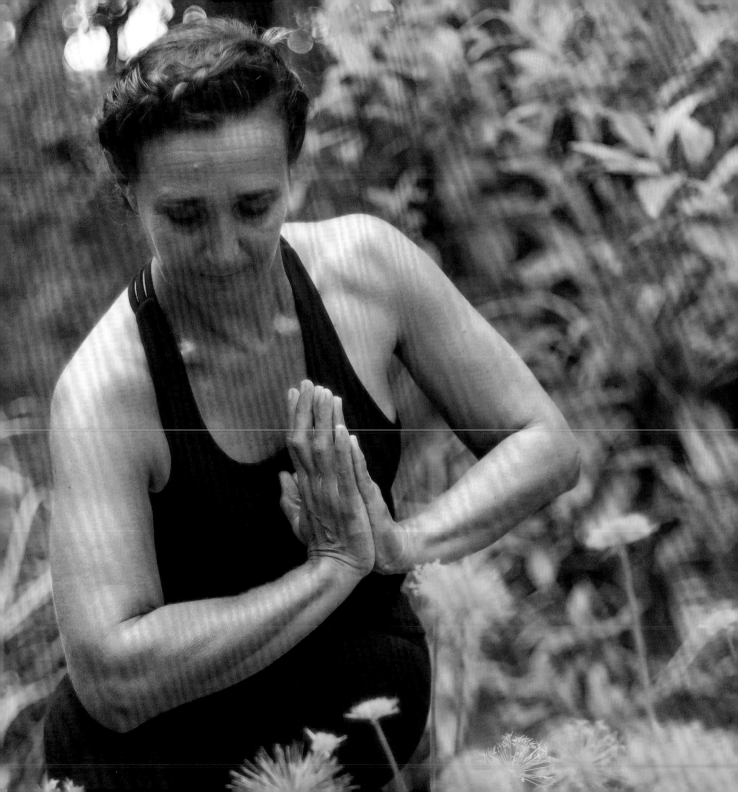

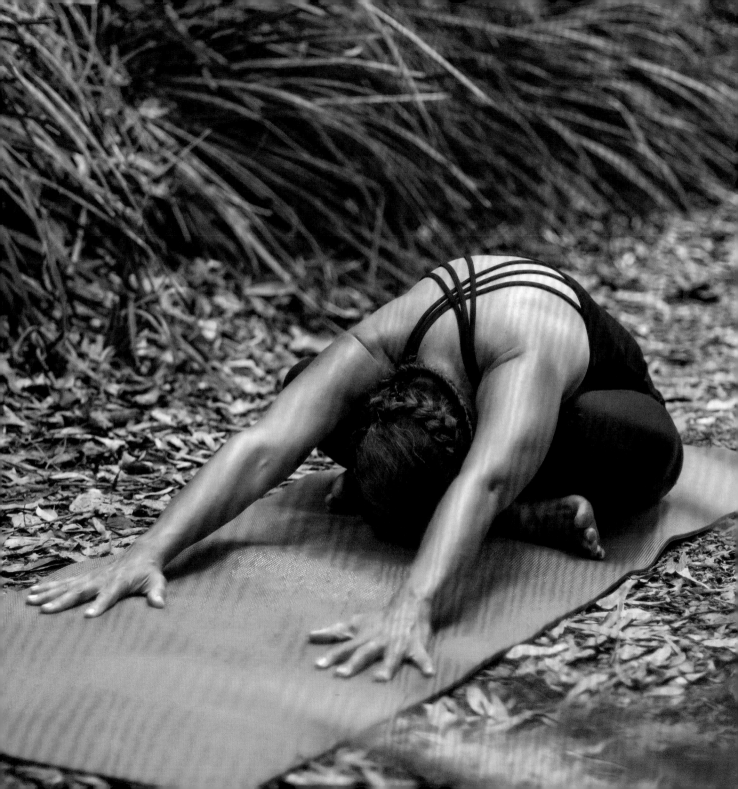

I EASY CROSS-LEGGED SEAT

OPEN
STRETCH
TONE
CALM

Come into a comfortable seated position crossing the legs at the shins.

Walk your hands out in front of you until the spine is extended and your chest is reaching towards the ground.

Release your head towards the ground.

Breathe here feeling the skin on the back of the body stretching.

Notice how one buttock is being stretched more than the other.

Hold the pose for 10 to 15 breaths.

Come up and change the cross of the shins so the other shin is in front.

When you are ready, come up and sit for a few moments feeling the body and mind calm and restored.

Benefits

Easy Cross-Legged Seat opens the outer hips.

It stretches the back of the body.

Tones the kidneys.

Calms the mind.

Lowers blood pressure because the head is below the heart.

Variations

Place your forehead on a block for extra support and to promote relaxation.

Place blocks under your thighs, if your knees don't easily relax to the floor.

| DOWN DOG POSE

Start in Child pose.

Reach your arms out in front of you spreading your fingers wide, the crease line of your wrist lined up with the end of your mat.

Tuck your toes under and, as you exhale, lift your buttocks towards the sky. If you're tight in the hamstrings, bend your knees.

If your spine is rounding and you feel too much weight in your arms, bend your knees more.

It should feel like you're pushing your hands away from the ground, extending your sitting bones (the point where your buttocks meet your leg) to the sky.

Feel the length in your spine and the space in between each vertebra.

On your next exhalation, come down and rest in Child pose.

Benefits

Down Dog stretches and lengthens the spine.

The head is lower than the heart so the nervous system relaxes.

It opens the hamstrings.

Releases the shoulders.

Strengthens the wrists and forearms.

It brings awareness to your breath and facilitates better breathing.

It challenges you to go beyond limitations; as you hold the pose and the arms get tired, staying there that little bit longer pushes you to the edge of your perceived boundaries.

Variations

Come into half dog, resting on your knees and walk your hands as far forward as possible so your torso is extended and the spine is lengthened. Breathe deeply feeling the stretch in the armpits. (See modifications p.291)

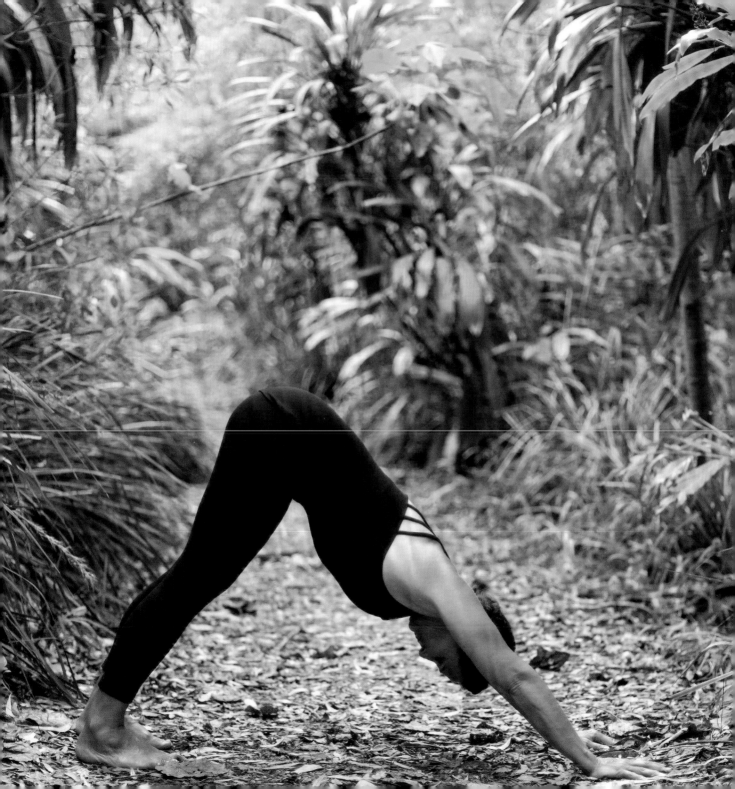

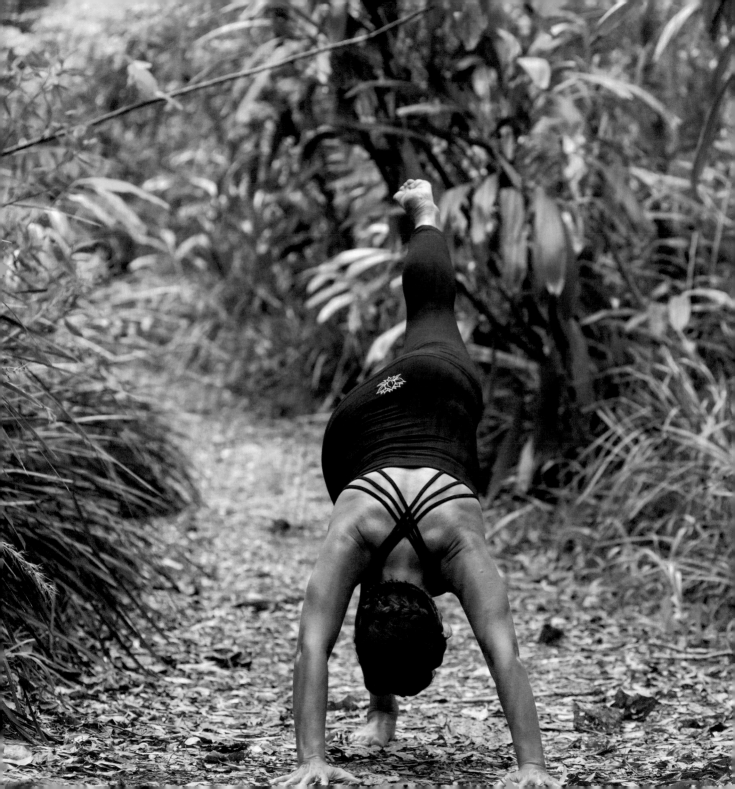

| ONE POINT POSE

Start in Down Dog pose.

Feel the weight spread evenly between the hands and feet.

Shift the weight to the left foot.

Exhale and raise the right leg into the air.

Lift the leg higher than hip height while keeping the knee facing towards the floor.

Feel the stretch in your left Achilles and calf muscle.

Keep your ribs from flaring out by engaging your abdominal muscles and feeling the front ribs coming closer together on exhalation.

Hold here for 5 breaths.

Lower the leg and repeat on the other side.

Complete the pose by returning to Down Dog.

Benefits

One Point pose develops strength and stamina.

It strengthens the arms, upper back and wrists.

It stretches the extended leg hip flexor.

Stretches the Achilles tendon and calf muscle.

Engages the hamstring of the lifted leg.

Variations

Bend the lifted leg at the knee.

Open the hip to the side of the lifted leg.

| LOW LUNGE POSE

Start in Down Dog pose.

Step your right foot far enough forward in between your hands so that the heel of your front foot is lined up with the heels of both hands.

Bring your torso into an upright position, keeping your hands on your hips.

Check to make sure your knee is directly over your ankle in a stacked position.

Raise your arms into the air and bring the palms to touch.

Keep the shoulders relaxed and gaze straight ahead.

Deepen the bend in the knee to feel the stretch in the hip flexor of the left leg.

Open the chest and breathe deeply.

Hold here for 5 to 10 breaths.

Bring the hands back down to either side of the right foot and step back into Down Dog.

Repeat on the other side.

Finish the second side in Down Dog pose.

Benefits

Low Lunge creates a deep stretch for the hip flexor.

It opens the chest and armpits facilitating drainage of the lymph system.

Strengthens the knee of the front leg.

Opens the front of the body from the pubic bone to the sternum.

A stimulating posture.

Variations

Bring the torso upright keeping the hands on the hips.

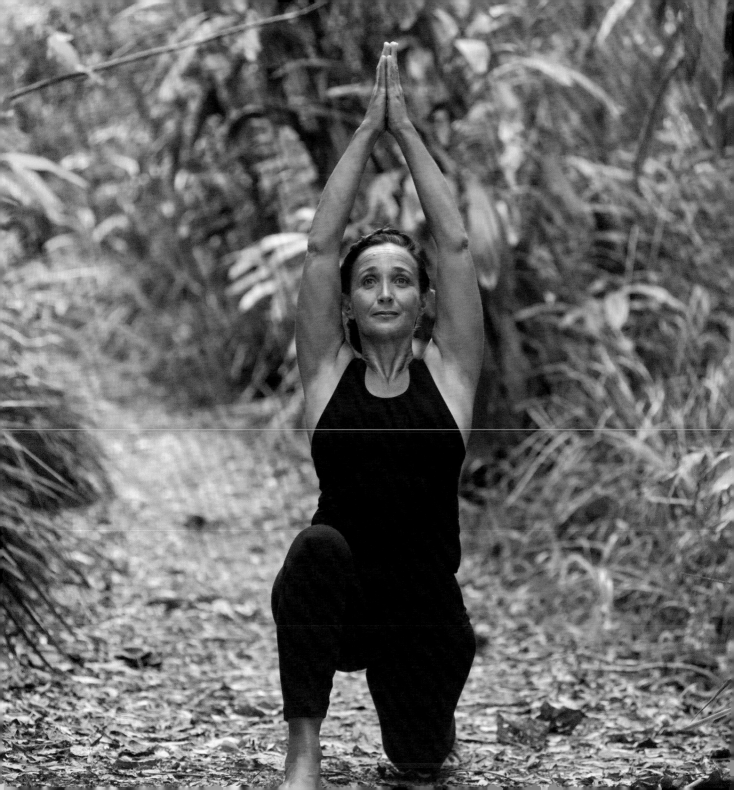

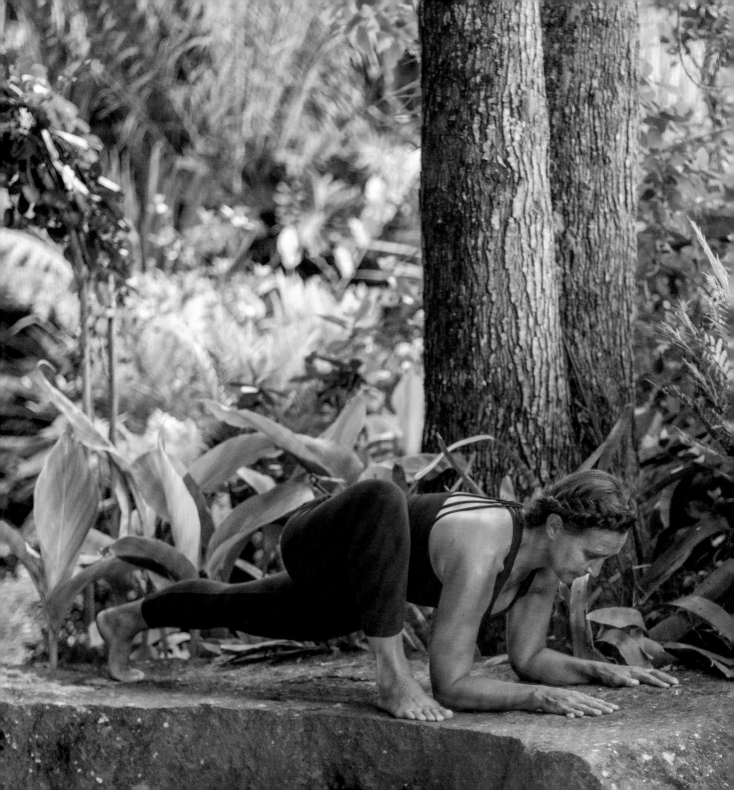

| LIZARD POSE

Start in Down Dog pose.

Step your right foot far enough forward in between your hands so that the heel of your front foot is lined up with the heels of both hands.

Turn your right foot slightly out to the side and place both hands on the inside of your right foot, then lower onto your forearms.

Keep the spine extended, feeling the length from your tailbone to your crown.

Squeeze your inner right thigh, pressing it against the right side of the torso.

Extend the back of your neck.

Feel the stretch in the front of the left groin.

Hold here for 5 to 10 breaths.

Step back into Down Dog.

Repeat on the other side.

Benefits

Lizard pose creates a deep stretch for your left hip flexor.

It's a good stretch for the back of your body.

It tones the kidney and adrenals.

Works your inner thigh muscles.

Opens and releases your chest, shoulders and neck.

Variations

Stay on your hands and keep your arms straight, if you can't easily reach the ground to rest on your forearms.

Bring your forearms onto a block.

| CRESCENT POSE

Stand at the top of your mat in Mountain pose, big toes touching, heels slightly apart. (You can find instructions for Mountain pose in the Vata sequence p.171)

Take a big step back with your left leg and face towards the left side of your mat.

Line up your right heel with the middle arch of your left foot.

Bend your front knee placing your hands on your hips.

Stack your front knee over your ankle.

Look down over your front knee and make sure you can still see all five toes and the top half of your front foot. (If you can't, you've bent your knee too much.)

Check to make sure your front knee isn't rolling in or out.

Turn in your back hip and foot to keep the front knee tracking over the ankle.

Slide your left hand down your left leg and raise your right arm, lean laterally to the left feeling a stretch in the right side of your ribcage.

Take 5 deep breaths here.

On your next exhalation, straighten the front leg.

Turn both feet to the center.

Repeat on the other side.

EXPAND
POWER
STAMINA
BREATHE

Benefits

Crescent posture builds strength and stamina.

It strengthens the knee joint and powers up the front thigh.

Facilitates deep breathing in the chest.

Strengthens the upper body.

Opens the hip flexor of the back leg and the muscles responsible for side bending.

Variations

Line up the front heel with the back heel, if your hips are tight.

Decrease the bend in the front knee, if the posture feels too strong or there is strain in your knee joint.

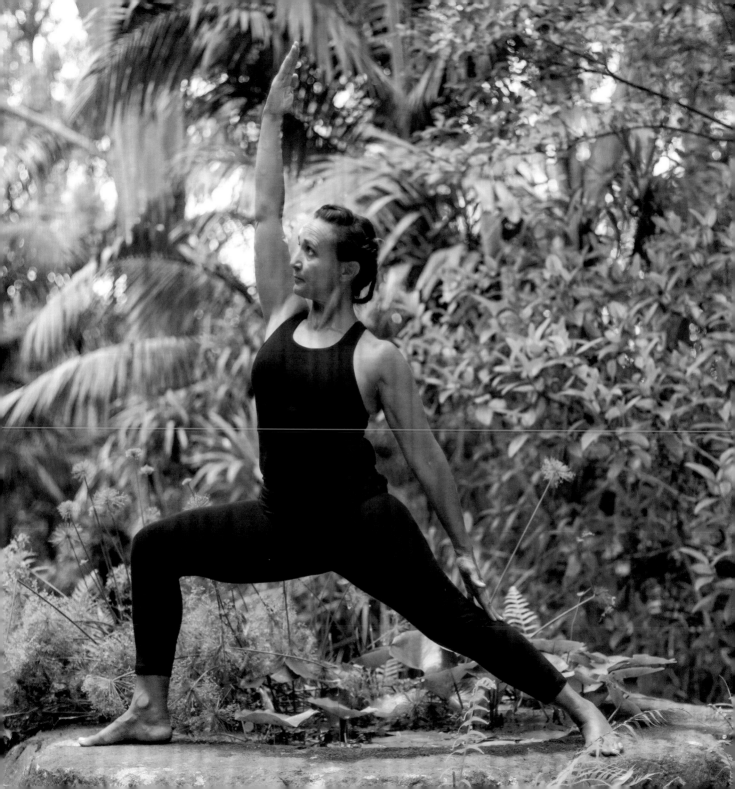

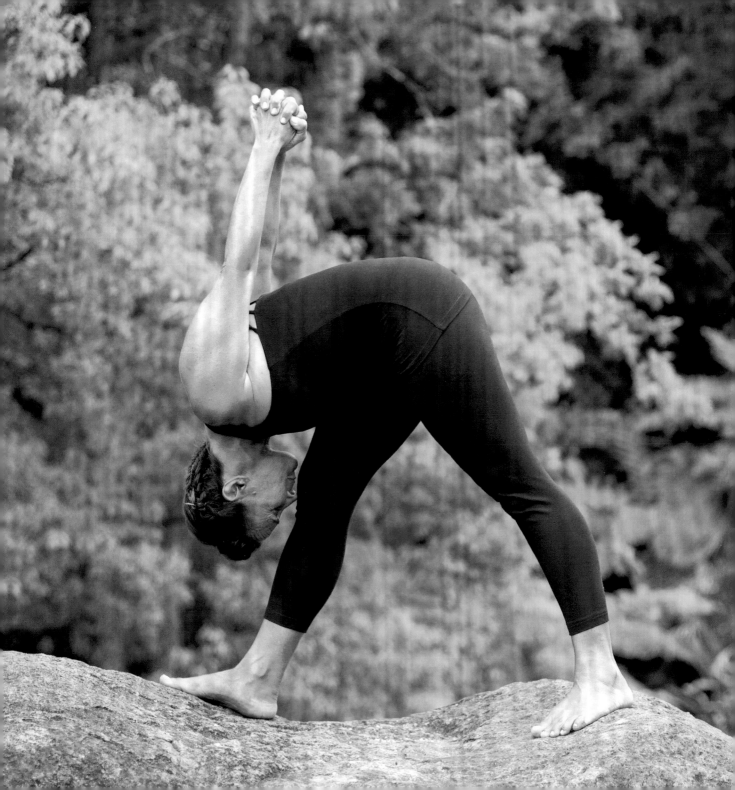

| TRIANGLE FORWARD BEND

Stand at the top of your mat in Mountain pose, big toes touching, heels slightly apart.

Take a medium step back with your left leg keeping both hips facing the front of the mat.

Interlace your fingers behind your back.

Inhale and lift your chest towards the sky.

As you exhale, fold forward at the hip crease, extending the spine until your belly and your front thigh meet.

Feel the clasped hands reaching over your head.

Bend the front knee slightly if the hamstring is tight.

Take 5 to 10 deep breaths.

Exhaling, ground down into your feet and bring your torso upright.

Inhaling, release the grip and clasp your hands the other way so the opposite fingers intertwine.

Step the left foot to the top of the mat and repeat on the other side.

Benefits

Triangle Forward Bend creates a deep stretch in the front hamstring.

The connection between the front thigh and the belly massages the internal organs.

Clasping the hands opens the shoulders.

A calming and cooling pose.

Variations

Fold the torso halfway, feeling length in the spine from the hips to the crown of the head. The back of the neck stays long as you gaze down. (This is referred to as a table top position.)

Bend the front knee, if your hamstring is tight.

| FAN POSE

Benefits

Fan pose is an inner thigh and hamstring stretch.

Your head is below your heart so it lowers your blood pressure and calms the mind.

It harmonizes the pineal, pituitary and thyroid glands.

Releases the head and the neck.

Strengthens the ankles.

Calms the nervous system.

Cools the body.

Variations

Place your hands on blocks underneath your shoulders, if you feel like you are rounding in your lower or upper back.

Bend your knees, if you feel tight in your hamstrings.

If your head easily touches the floor, bring your feet closer towards each other.

If your head does not easily touch the ground, bring your feet wider apart.

Step the feet wide apart, toes facing forward, edges of the feet lined up with the edges of the mat.

Place your hands on your hips, inhale and open the chest towards the sky.

As you exhale, hinge at the hips and fold far enough forward so that your head is reaching towards the ground.

Lengthen your spine and roll your thighs inwards creating space in the lower back.

Lift the thigh muscles up towards the hips.

Hold here for 10 breaths.

Complete your last exhalation and bring the torso upright on the next inhalation.

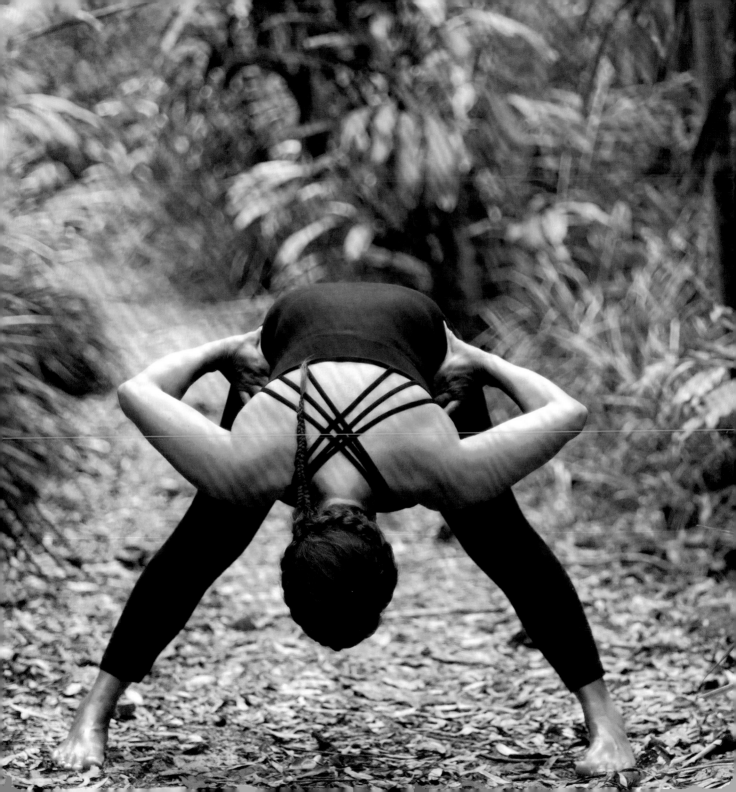

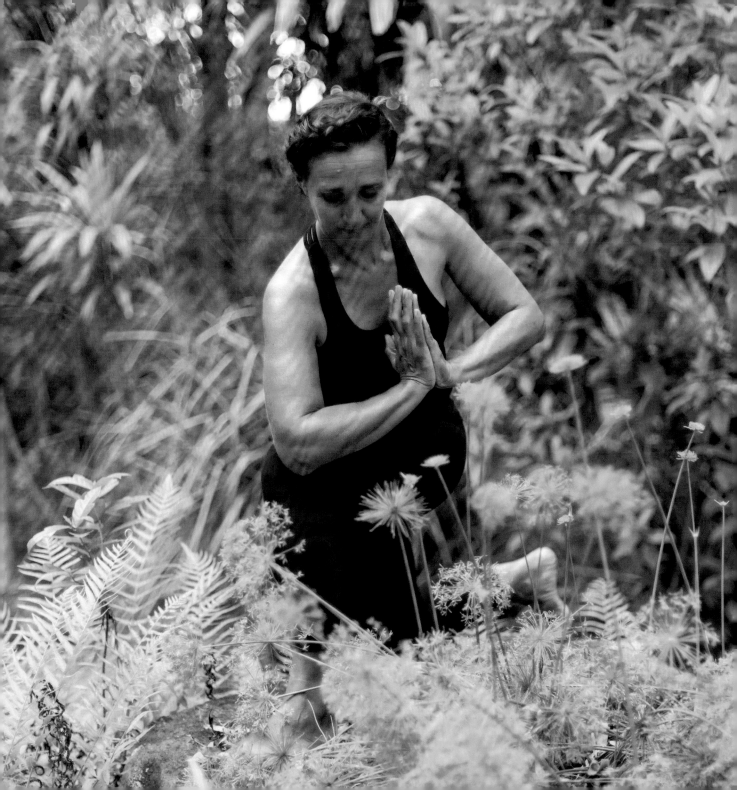

| REVOLVED RIGHT ANGLE POSE

Come onto your hands and knees.

Step your left foot in between your hands and bring your torso upright so you are in the Low Lunge position.

Check to make sure your front knee is stacked over your ankle and that your back hip and back knee are in line.

As you move into the pose, your hip will come slightly forward out of alignment.

Place your hands in prayer position at your heart.

Inhale and turn your torso to the left.

Exhale and place your upper right arm against your outer left thigh.

The more you lever your upper arm against your outer thigh, the more deeply you can twist.

Take 5 deep breaths here twisting deeper on the inhalation and resting in place on the exhalation.

Turn back to center on your final exhalation.

Return to your hands and knees and repeat on the other side.

Benefits

Revolved Right Angle is an outer hip stretch.

The deep twist massages the internal organs.

It brings nourishment into the discs between the vertebrae of your spine.

Stretches the groin and hip flexors.

Strengthens the knee of the front leg.

Brings the breath into areas it wouldn't normally reach.

Variations

Keep the hands in prayer position and straighten the back leg lifting the back knee off the ground.

| CHILD POSE

CALM
NEUTRAL
REST
REPLENISH

Start on your hands and knees.

Exhaling, send your buttocks back to your heels.

Rest your chest to your thighs, forehead on the ground and have your hands reaching out in front.

Breathe here, feeling the belly pressed against the thighs and the skin on the back of the body stretching.

Benefits

Child pose is a neutral position for your spine.

Your head is below your heart, which lowers your blood pressure.

It massages the internal organs.

It's nourishing for the kidneys and adrenals, because the breath is directed towards the back of the body.

A great resting posture.

Variations

Place a block under your forehead, if your head does not easily touch the floor.

Place a bolster behind your knees to create more space, if you are tight in your thighs.

Relax the arms alongside the body to make the pose more passive.

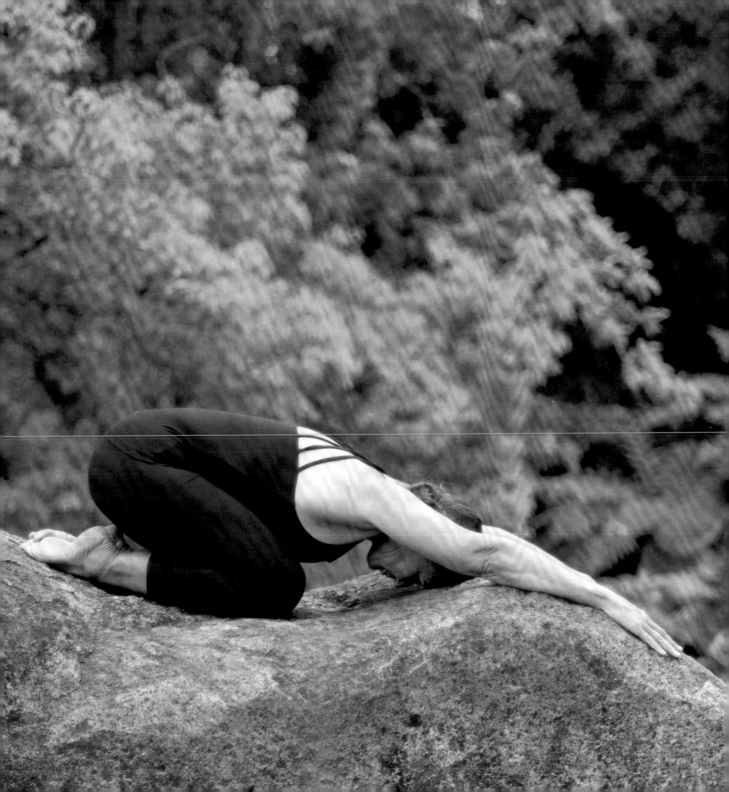

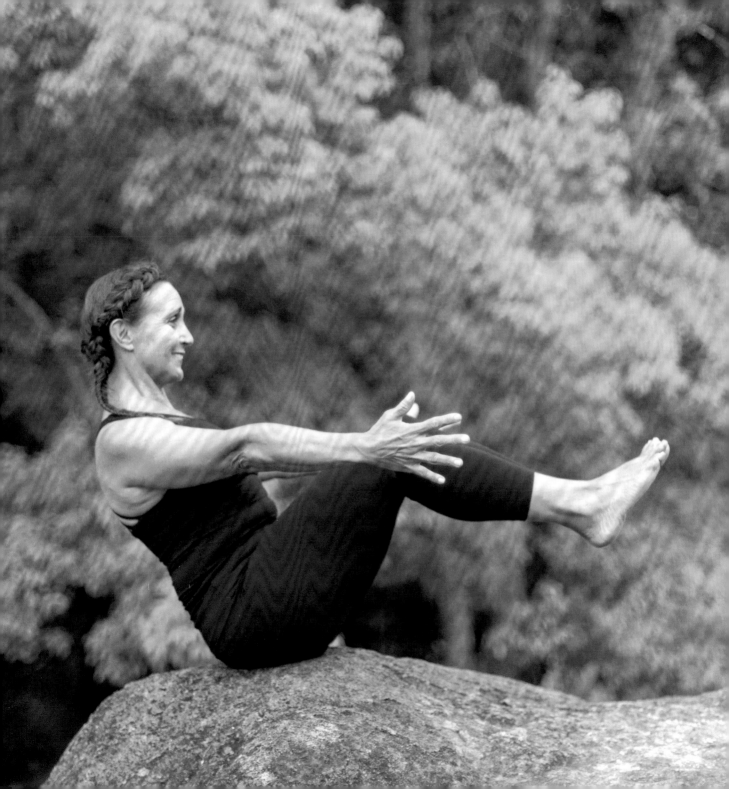

| BOAT POSE

BUILD
HEAT
TONE
STAMINA

Sit on your buttocks.

Bend the knees and have the feet flat on the ground and slightly out in front of you.

Place your hands behind your knees, shift the weight back to just behind your sitting bones and come to the tips of your toes.

Lift the feet off the floor keeping the knees bent.

Depending on your balance and strength, you can either have the feet lower than the knees or lift the feet so they line up with the knees.

Breathe here feeling the core muscles engaged.

Lower the feet back to the ground and place your hands on the ground behind you.

Benefits

Boat pose strengthens the core.

It builds heat.

Tones the abdominals.

Engages the thigh muscles.

An effective counter pose to the back bends.

Variations

Take hold of the backs of the thighs with the hands.

Keep feet lower than knees.

Straighten the legs. (This is more challenging.)

I LOCUST POSE

Lie on your belly, forehead pressing into the ground, arms relaxed alongside the body with your thighs, knees and toes all facing down.

Interlace your fingers at the small of your back.

On your next inhalation, lift your feet, legs, upper chest, arms and head off the ground.

Activate the inner thighs and lift them towards the sky while relaxing the buttocks.

Open through the front of the chest, keeping the bottom of your ribs, entire abdomen and pubic bone on the ground.

Keep your neck in line with your spine.

Gaze forwards.

Take 5 to 10 breaths here.

Come down, turn your head to one side and relax.

Benefits

Locust pose works the muscles on either side of the spine, toning the kidneys and adrenals.

It massages the internal organs.

Engages the breath in your upper chest.

Releases the lower back, while working the hamstrings.

Opens the shoulders.

An energizing, stimulating pose.

Variations

Move on the breath, inhaling and lifting into the pose, exhaling and relaxing back down.

Unclasp the hands and reach the arms alongside the torso, your palms facing down.

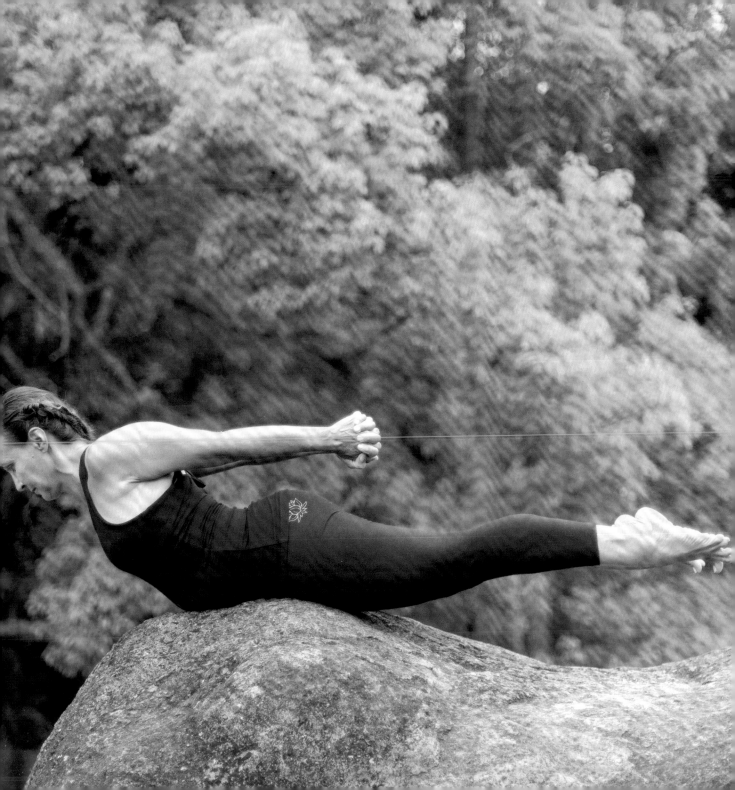

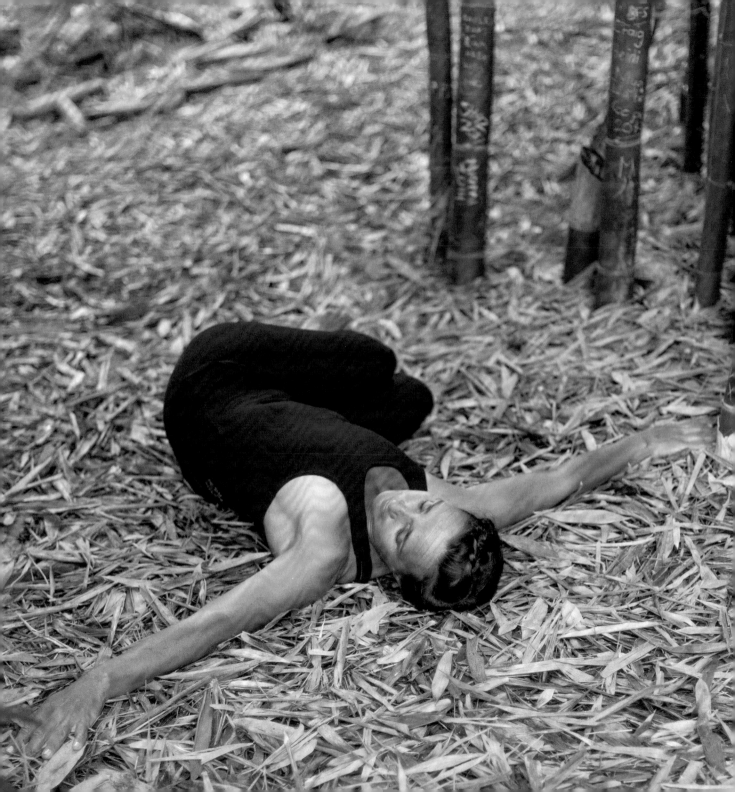

| MALTESE TWIST POSE

Lie on your back with your knees bent and feet flat on the ground.

Have your feet slightly in front of your knees and hip-width apart.

Inhaling, lift your hips, shifting them a few inches to the right side.

Exhaling, lift the knees so they are close to your chest.

Inhaling, lower the knees to the left side.

Slightly arch your lower back to create length in your spine.

Line up your feet with your knees so they form a right angle.

Feel both sides of the body lengthening as the chest rotates open.

Breathe here for 5 to 10 rounds.

On your next exhalation, come back to center placing your feet on the ground slightly forward of your knees.

Repeat on the other side.

Benefits

The Maltese Twist releases the lower back.

It stretches your outer hip.

Opens the ribcage.

Opens the breath.

Opens the shoulders.

A relaxing, cooling and calming posture.

Variations

If your right shoulder doesn't touch the ground, bend your right elbow and rest your hand on the right side of your ribcage.

| SAGE POSE

Sit on your buttocks with both legs extended out in front of you.

Bend you right knee and cross your right foot over your left leg. (The right foot is facing the same direction as your extended leg and is flat on the ground.)

Place your right hand on the ground behind you, the heel of your hand in line with the center of your spine and slightly away from the body.

Inhale and extend your left arm high into the air and then twist the upper body to the right, wrapping your upper left arm around your outer right thigh.

Exhale and relax.

Inhale and twist further making sure the movement for the twist is coming from the torso and not the head.

Gaze over your right shoulder.

Breathe deeply and hold for 5 breaths.

Turn back to center, unwind the legs and repeat the posture on the other side.

Benefits

Sage pose creates an outer hip stretch.

The deep twist massages the internal organs.

It brings nourishment into the discs between the vertebrae of your spine.

It provides a gentle hamstring stretch for the extended leg.

It's nourishing and calming for the nervous system.

It focuses the mind by bringing it to the breath.

Variations

Bring the upper left arm to the outside of the right thigh to deepen the twist.

Gaze over your left shoulder.

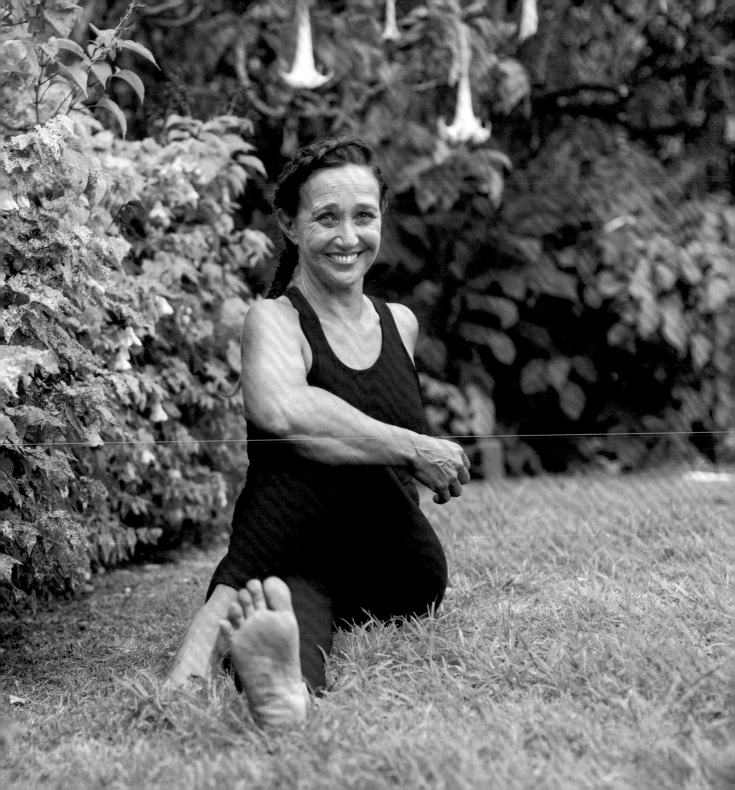

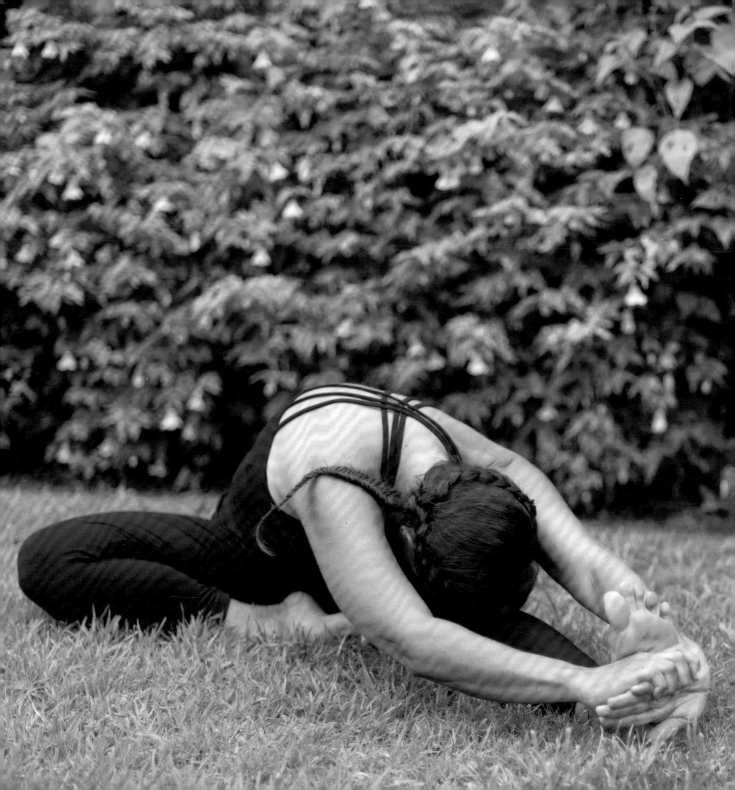

| HEAD TO KNEE POSE

LENGTHEN
RESTORE
SOOTHE
CALM

Sit on your buttocks with both legs extended out in front of you.

Bend the right knee and place the sole of the foot close to the groin on the inside of the left thigh.

Flex both feet, activating the extended leg, while keeping the knee facing towards the ceiling.

Inhaling, lengthen the spine and begin to fold forward from the hips.

Exhaling, reach the hands to either side of the leg.

Only take hold of the foot if your abdomen easily touches your thigh.

Most importantly, keep the chest open and breathe deeply.

On your next inhalation, return to the upright position and repeat the posture on the other side.

Benefits

Head to Knee pose is a great stretch for the hamstrings.

It opens the hips.

Stretches and tones the adrenals and kidneys.

A calming and relaxing posture.

Variations

Bend the knee of the extended leg if you feel pulling on your lower back or in your hamstrings and rest your abdomen on your thigh.
(See modifications p.296)

| REVOLVED HEAD TO KNEE POSE

TURN
LIFT
BROADEN
BREATHE

Sit on your buttocks with both legs extended out in front of you.

Bend the right knee and place the sole of the foot close to the groin on the inside of the left thigh.

Flex both feet, activating the extended leg while keeping the knee facing towards the ceiling.

Turn your torso so that you can slide the left forearm on the ground along the inside thigh of the left leg.

Take hold of the inside of your left foot.

Reach the right arm over your head with the intention of grasping the outside of your right foot.

Gently twist the spine rolling the right side of the chest towards the ceiling.

Stay here for 5 to 10 breaths, breathing deeply.

Inhale and bring the torso upright.

Stay here for a few minutes until you feel your energy balancing.

Repeat on the other side.

Benefits

Revolved Head to Knee pose is a deep stretch for the kidneys.

It's a lateral stretch that opens the ribcage and facilitates deep breathing.

It also provides a strong inner thigh stretch on the extended leg.

It releases pent-up energy.

A rejuvenating and balancing pose.

Variations

Rest your lower arm on a block, bringing the ground to you.

Reach your arm alongside your ear.

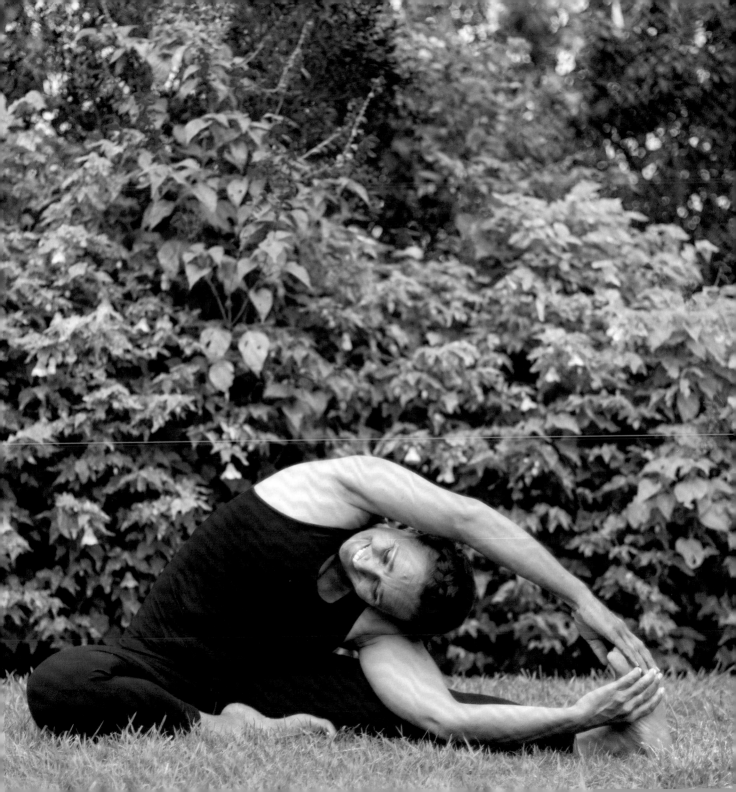

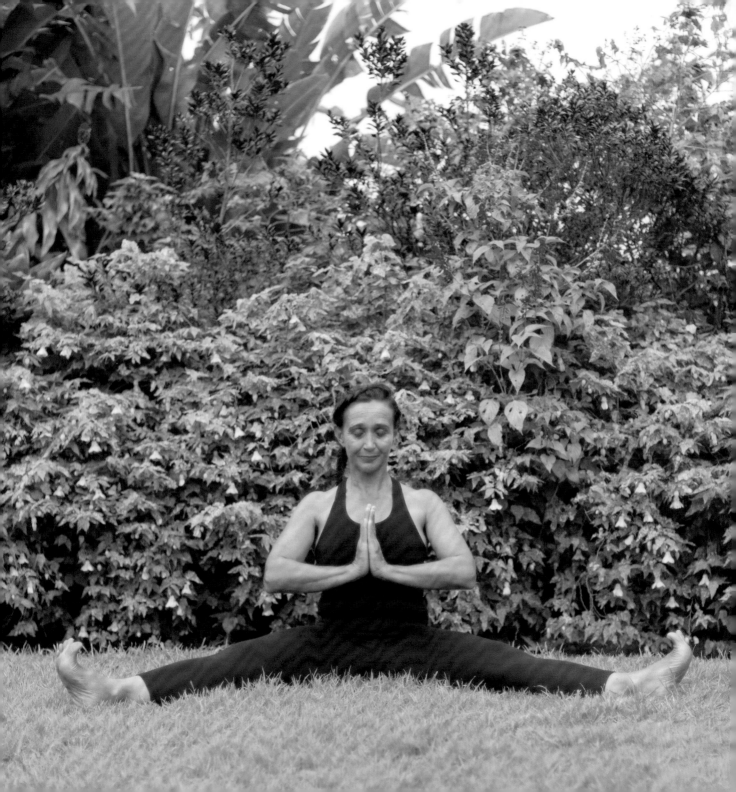

| WIDE ANGLE SEATED POSE

Sit on the center of the sitting bones, spine long, legs extended forward and parallel.

Open both legs out to the side.

Flex the feet, activating the legs so your toes and knees point up towards the ceiling.

Open through the chest and breathe deeply.

Keep the neck long and chin level to the floor.

Bring the hands into prayer position and close the eyes.

Hold here for 5 to 10 breaths.

To come out of the posture, place the palms flat on the ground behind you, lean back and scissor the legs back to parallel.

Benefits

Wide Angle Seated Pose is an inner thigh and hamstring stretch.

It engages the abdominal and back muscles.

A calming and centering pose.

Variations

Sit on a blanket, if you are rounding in your lower spine, bringing the hips higher than the thighs.

Bend the knees, if you feel tension in your hamstrings.

| COW FACE POSE

Come onto your hands and knees.

Tuck the right knee in behind the left knee and sit back between your feet with your buttocks on the floor so that the shins and feet flare out to the side.

Your left thigh will be crossed over your right.

Your knees are stacked on top of each other.

The feet are equidistant from the buttocks.

Lengthen the spine and open the chest.

Place one hand on top of the other extending your thumbs out to the side and resting your hands on your knee.

Close the eyes and breathe deeply for 5 to 10 breaths.

Come back on to your hands and knees and change sides.

Benefits

Cow Face is a deep outer thigh stretch.

It provides a stretch for the buttocks.

The hand position facilitates deep relaxation.

A calming, nurturing pose.

Variations

Extend the bottom leg, if the thighs are tight.

Sit on a block, if the lower back rounds.

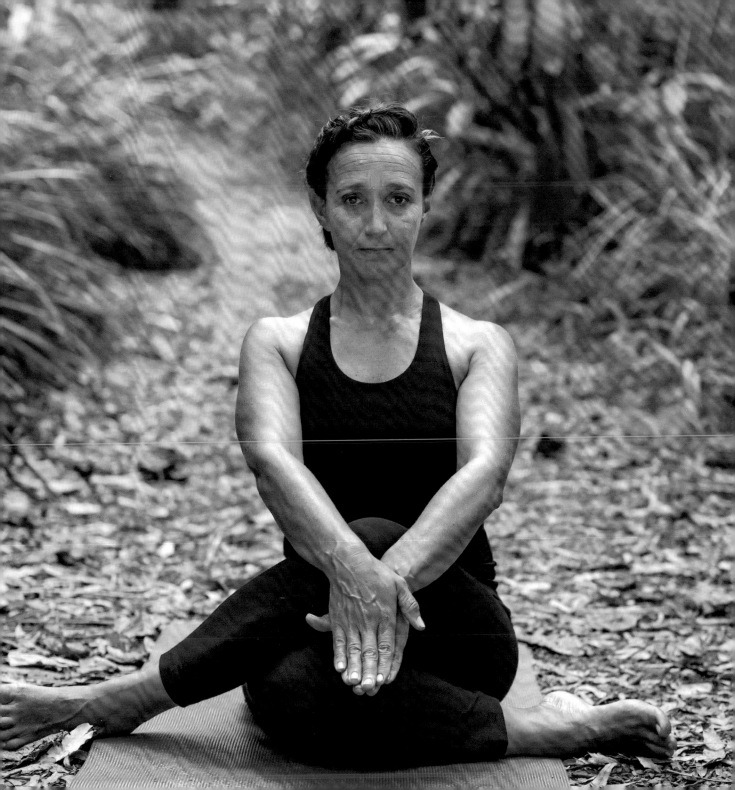

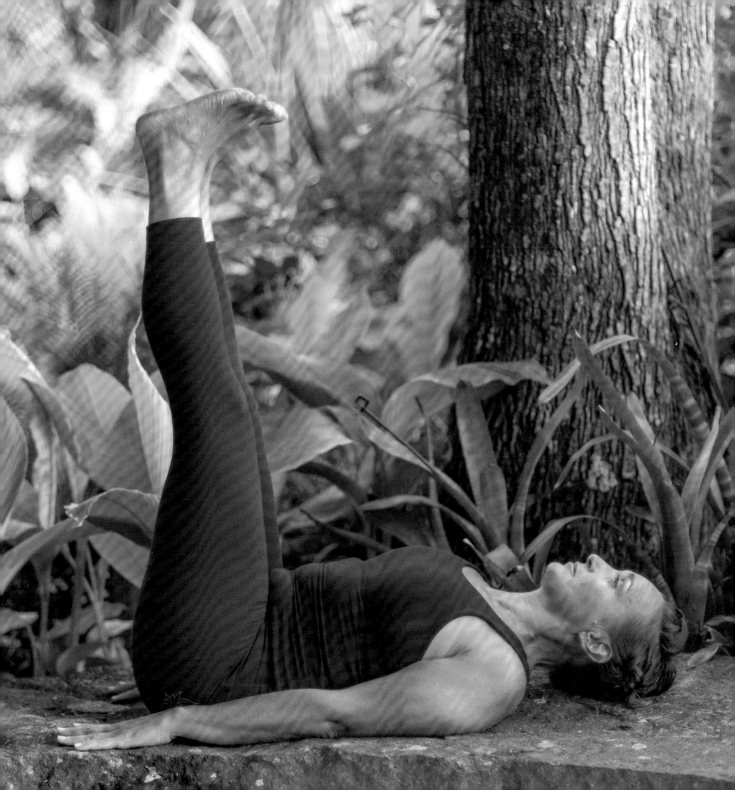

| INVERTED LEG POSE

INVERT
LOWER
REDUCE
SUPPORT

Lie on your back with your knees bent and feet flat on the floor beneath you.

Exhaling, draw both knees to your chest.

Inhale and extend your feet to the sky.

Rest your arms alongside your body.

Hold here for 10 to 15 breaths.

Your abdominals will be gently engaged.

To finish, exhale and bend the knees back into the chest.

Lower the feet to the floor.

Rest here for a moment knees touching and feet wide apart.

Benefits

Inverted Leg posture reduces swelling in your feet and legs and promotes some fluid drainage.

It helps prevent varicose veins.

It can lower your blood pressure.

Gently works the abdominal muscles.

It's soothing for the nervous system.

Variations

Bend the knees, if the hamstrings are tight.

Rest your legs up a wall.

Place a block under your lower back to lift the pelvis a bit more and increase the fluid drainage.

| RECLINING BUDDHA POSE

Lie on your back, bending the knees and bringing the soles of the feet together.

The feet can be close to the groin or further away depending on what's comfortable.

Close your eyes and place your hands on your belly.

Breathe deeply and relax for 20 breaths.

Benefits

Reclining Buddha is a deep inner thigh stretch.

It increases circulation to your pelvis.

It supports your reproductive and hormonal system.

A calming and grounding posture.

Variations

Place blocks under the thighs if the hips are tight.

If it's uncomfortable in the lower back to lie flat on the ground, place a bolster in the vertical position at the base of the thoracic spine. Recline over it, so that your head and upper chest are resting on the bolster. This also opens the chest and facilitates deep breathing.

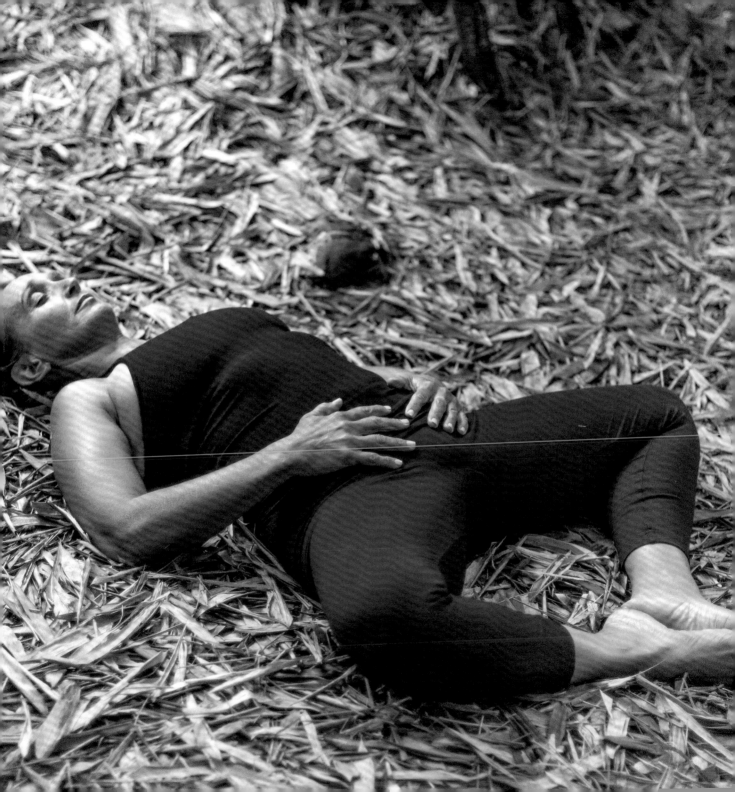

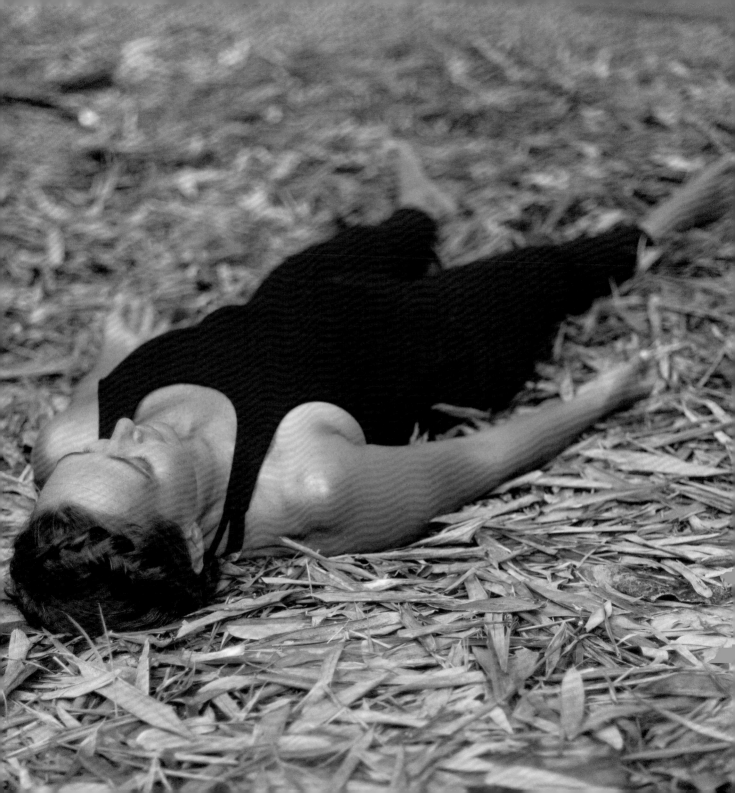

| CORPSE POSE

Lie on your back.

Have your arms and legs slightly away from the body, palms facing upwards, feet relaxed and open.

Turn the head gently from side to side until it rests in the center.

If your chin juts up towards the sky, place a blanket underneath your head.

Relax completely.

Don't worry about the breath or what the body is doing.

Feel how effortless it is to lie here.

Stay here for at least 5 minutes.

When you are ready, roll to one side and come up.

Benefits

This is the most important posture in the sequence. Missing this posture is like making a meal and then deciding not to eat it.

All the nourishing and healing benefits of the practice are integrated in this posture.

The relaxed part of the nervous system is engaged.

The body releases and relaxes at a cellular level.

The glandular system is replenished.

The alpha and theta brainwaves are dominant and the mind relaxes.

Variations

Place a bolster under your knees, if there is pressure in your lower back.

Place an inch-thick folded blanket under the head, if there is any tension in the neck.

Place an eye pillow over your eyes, if you have an active mind.

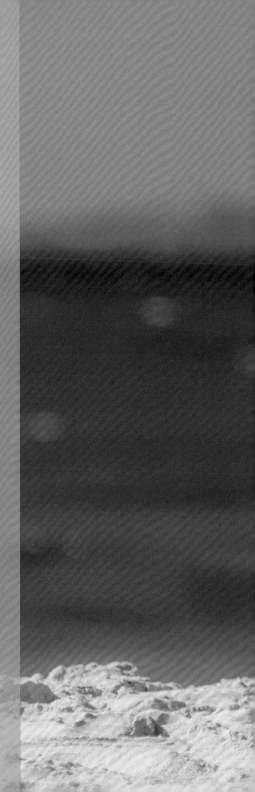

KAPHAS ARE INCREDIBLY LOVING. THEY FORGIVE EASILY AND LIKE HAVING FUN.

INTENTION

MAY I FEEL ENERGIZED,
MOTIVATED AND INSPIRED

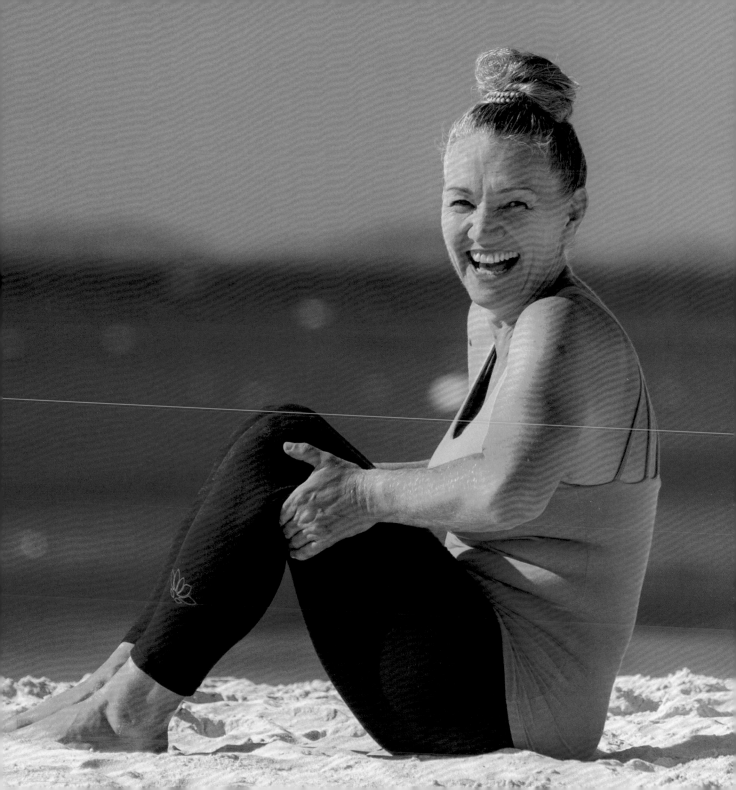

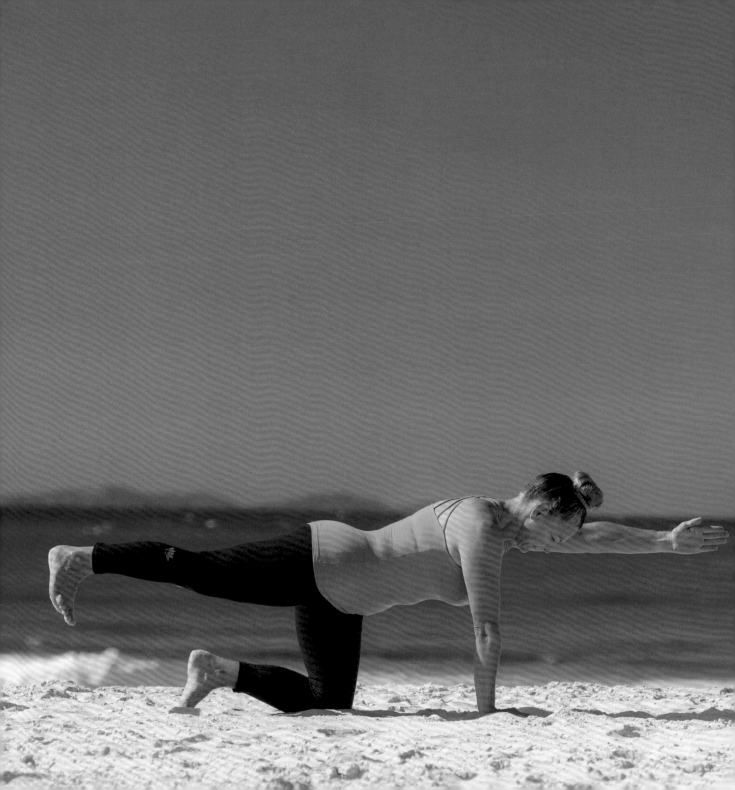

| TIGER POSE

Come onto your hands and knees.

Place your hands underneath your shoulders and your knees underneath your hips.

Inhale and lengthen the spine.

Exhaling, gently raise your right arm into the air, extending the arm out to the front.

Extend your left leg behind you and inhale deeply.

Engage your abdominals, rolling your left thigh down, left knee facing the ground.

Feel your inner thighs working towards each other.

Slowly lower your right hand and left leg, returning to resting on your hands and knees.

Repeat on the other side, raising the opposite arm and leg.

Benefits

Tiger pose is excellent for strengthening the abdominals.

It works with left and right coordination balancing the nervous system.

It works the hamstrings.

Strengthens the upper arms and wrists.

Heats and energizes the body.

Starting with this pose focuses the mind and challenges you to be present.

Variations

If your wrists are weak, place your weight on your forearms instead of your hands.

If your knees are sensitive, place a blanket underneath your knees.

| DOWN DOG POSE

Start in Child pose.

Reach your arms out in front of you spreading your fingers wide, the crease line of your wrist lined up with the end of your mat.

Tuck your toes under and, as you exhale, lift your buttocks towards the sky. If you're tight in the hamstrings, bend your knees.

If your spine is rounding and you feel too much weight in your arms, bend your knees more.

It should feel like you're pushing your hands away from the ground, extending your sitting bones (the point where your buttocks meet your leg) to the sky.

Feel the length in your spine and the space in between each vertebra.

On your next exhalation, come down and rest in Child pose.

Benefits

Down Dog stretches and lengthens the spine.

The head is lower than the heart so the nervous system relaxes.

It opens the hamstrings.

Releases the shoulders.

Strengthens the wrists and forearms.

It brings awareness to your breath and facilitates better breathing.

It challenges you to go beyond limitations; as you hold the pose and the arms get tired, staying there that little bit longer pushes you to the edge of your perceived boundaries.

Variations

Bend your knees if your hamstrings are tight or you feel pulling on your lower back.

Come into half dog, resting on your knees and walking your hands as far forward as possible so your torso is extended and the spine is lengthened. Breathe deeply feeling the stretch in the armpits. (See modifications p.291)

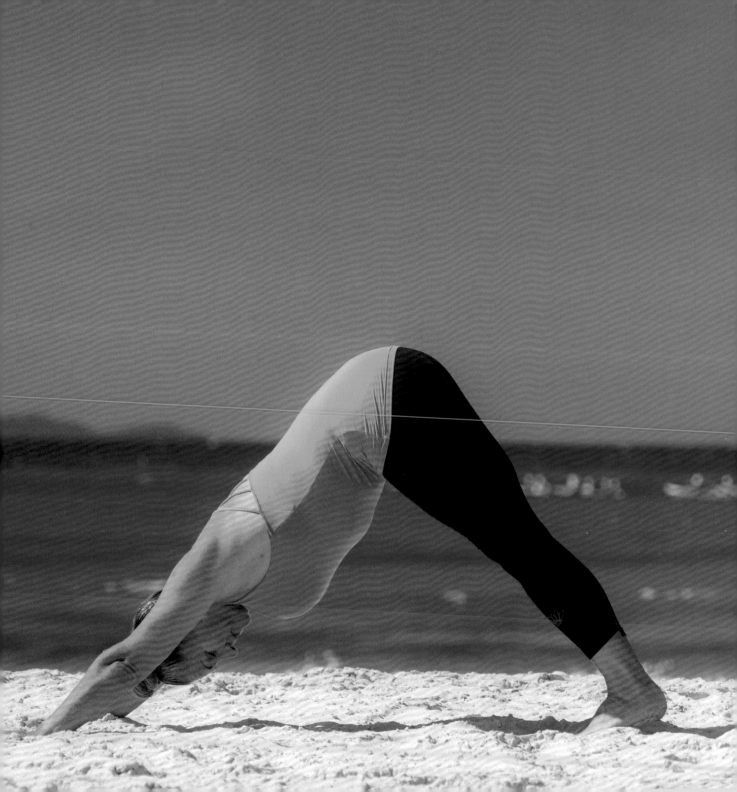

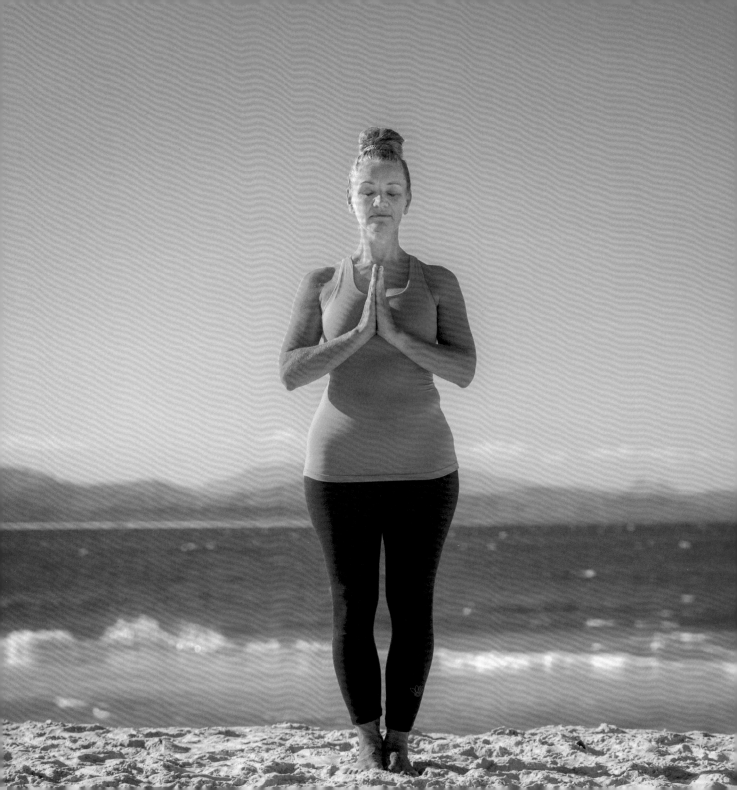

| MOUNTAIN POSE

SUPPORT
BALANCE
CALM
REST

Stand with the big toes touching and the heels slightly apart.

Feel the weight balanced between the four corners of the foot: the outer heel, little toe mound, big toe mound and inner heel.

Engage the thighs keeping the knees soft.

Feel your tailbone lengthening.

Create space between the top of your hipbones and the base of your ribcage.

Open the chest, relax the shoulders and keep the chin level.

Bring the hands into prayer position.

Benefits

Mountain pose is one of the safest positions for the spine.

The weight is balanced between both feet which supports the spine in maintaining its natural curves.

This means there is no significant strain in any part of the body.

This pose supports the body in bearing weight.

It facilitates easy and open breathing.

A calming posture.

Perfect resting pose between the standing postures.

Variations

Relax the arms alongside the body, slightly roll the upper arms out and the forearms in.

Interlace the fingers in front of the chest and raise the arms up over the head.

| MOON POSE

LEAN
OPEN
SUPPORT
ELIMINATE

Stand in Mountain pose, big toes touching, heels slightly apart.

Inhaling, raise your arms up, bringing your palms to touch.

Lifting and lengthening the torso, lean over to one side.

Breathe deeply into the stretch, keeping the belly firm.

Inhale and return to center.

Keeping the arms extended and the palms touching, lean to the other side and breathe deeply.

On your next inhalation, return back to center.

Lower the arms and rest in Mountain pose.

Benefits

Moon pose creates a lateral stretch with space between the intercostal muscles (the muscles in between the ribs).

It supports the kidneys and adrenals by bringing fresh blood and circulation into the area.

Increases the breath capacity in the chest area.

Supports the lymph system to eliminate waste.

Variations

If you are tight in the shoulders, bend at the elbows and keep the palms together as you lean to the side.

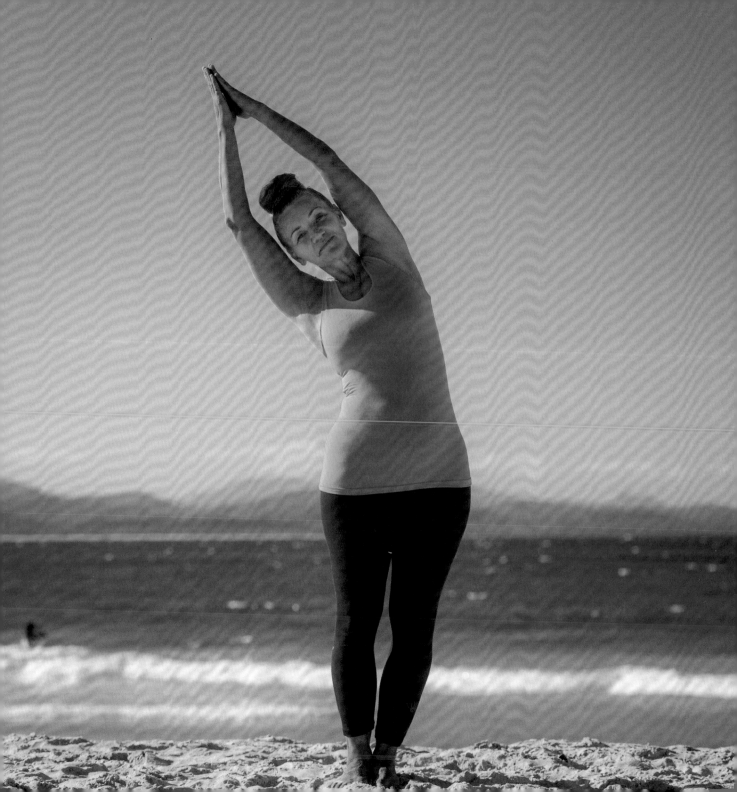

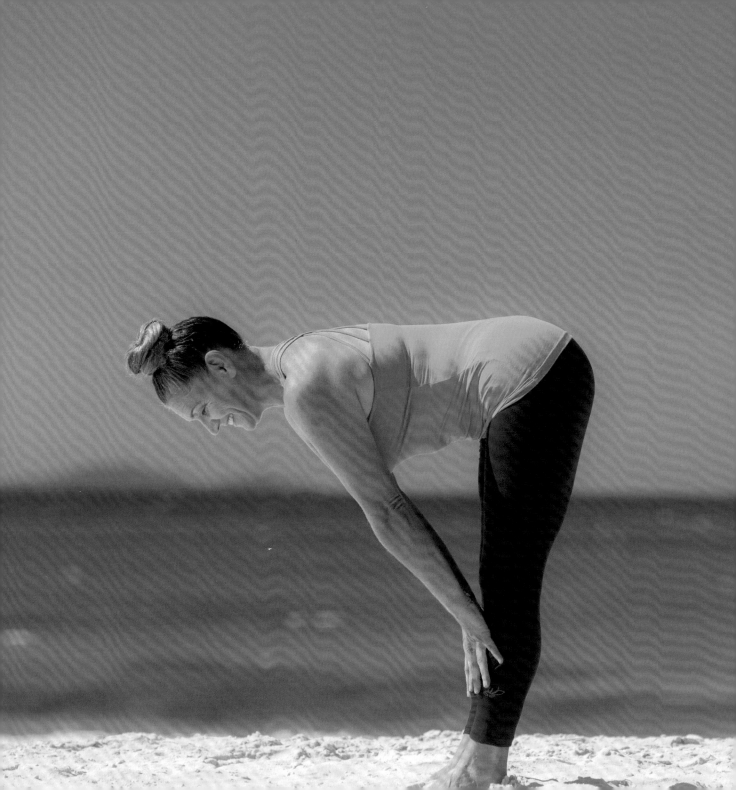

I PREPARE POSE

STRENGTH
LENGTHEN
FREEDOM
SMOOTHE

Stand at the top of your mat in Mountain pose, big toes touching, heels slightly apart.

Place your hands on your hips and take an inhalation.

Exhale and fold forward at the hip crease keeping your spine long and coming to a table top position (with a flat back).

If your hamstrings are tight or your lower back has a pulling sensation, bend your knees.

Place your hand on your shins.

Engage the thigh muscles. (You can do this whether your knees are bent or straight.)

Breathe fully and deeply into the chest.

Inhale and raise the torso, returning to Mountain pose.

Benefits

Prepare pose works both the abdominal muscles and the back muscles, developing core strength.

It opens the hamstrings and strengthens the thigh muscles.

Lengthens the spine, stretching the vertebrae.

Opens the chest so breathing is smoother and freer.

Variations

Place your hands on either your thighs or on blocks to bring the floor to you.
(See modifications p.292)

| PLANK POSE

Come onto your hands and knees.

Place your hands underneath your shoulders and your knees underneath your hips.

Extend one leg behind you and press the ball of the foot into the ground.

Extend the other leg back and feel your weight balanced between the hands and the balls of the feet.

Keep the body in one line.

Push the ground away and feel a slight round in the upper chest so the shoulders sit on the spine.

Feel how the core automatically engages.

Breathe deeply enjoying the warmth and power this pose generates.

Exhale and drop your knees to the ground.

Rest in Child pose.

Benefits

Plank strengthens the wrists, arms and shoulders.

It tones abdominals.

Builds strength and stamina.

Plank is a total body workout and heat-building pose.

Variations

Tiger pose.

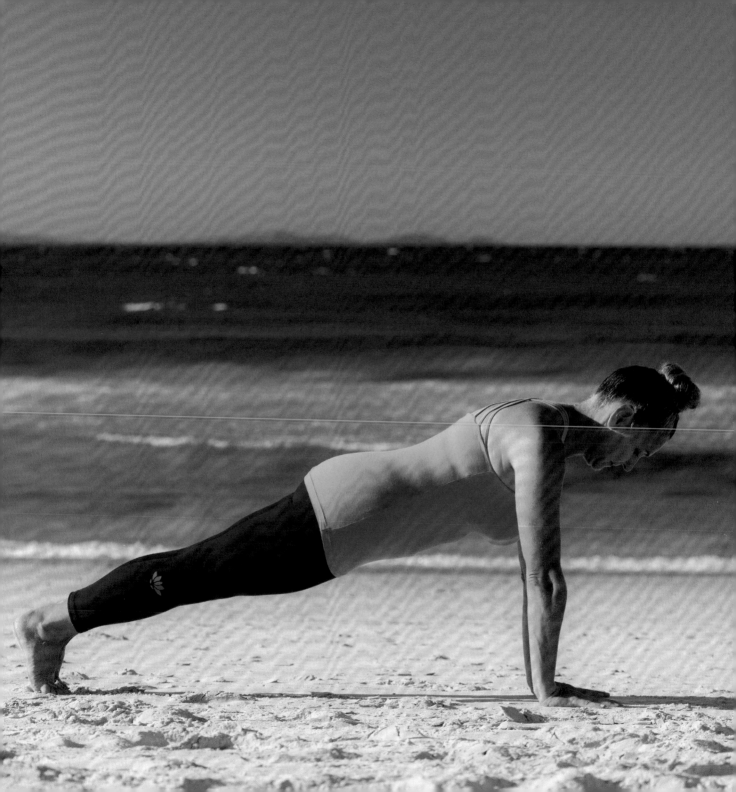

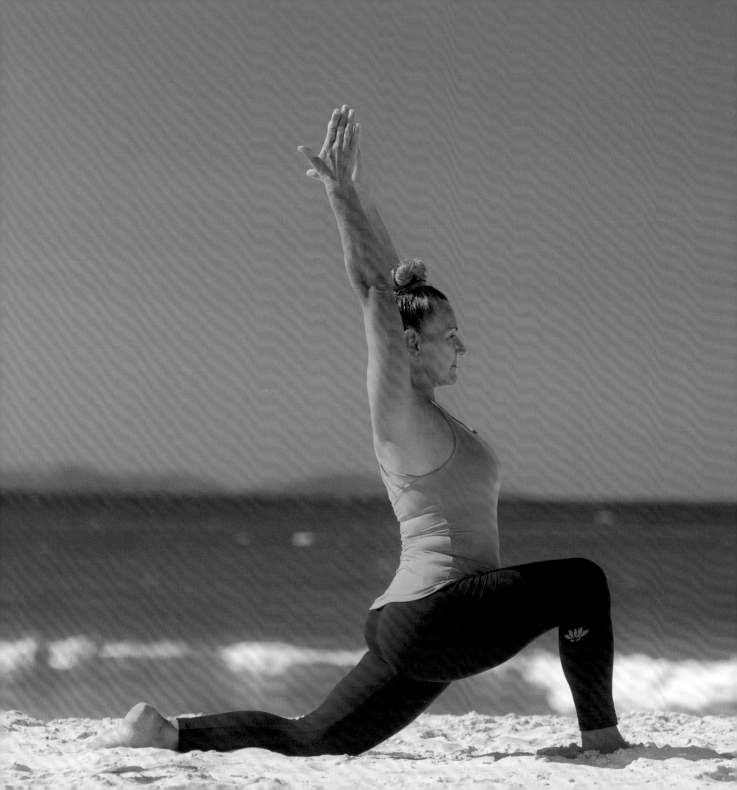

| LOW LUNGE

OPEN
STRETCH
TONE
DEEPEN

Start in Down Dog pose.

Step your right foot far enough forward in between your hands so that the heel of your front foot is lined up with the heels of both hands.

Bring your torso into an upright position, keeping your hands on your hips.

Check to make sure your knee is directly over your ankle in a stacked position.

Raise your arms into the air and have them shoulder distance apart.

Keep the shoulders relaxed and gaze straight ahead.

Deepen the bend in the knee to feel the stretch in the hip flexor of the left leg.

Open the chest and breathe deeply.

Hold here for 5 to 10 breaths.

Bring the hands back down to either side of the right foot and step back into Down Dog.

Repeat on the other side.

Finish the second side in Down Dog pose.

Benefits

Low Lunge creates a deep stretch for the hip flexor.

It opens the chest and armpits facilitating drainage of the lymph system.

Strengthens the knee of the front leg.

Opens the front of the body from the pubic bone to the sternum.

A stimulating posture.

Variations

Keep hands on the floor either side of your front foot and breathe deeply feeling your chest pressed against your thigh. A great massage for the internal organs.
(See modifications p.293)

| CHAIR POSE

STRENGTH
ENDURANCE
BROADEN
POWER

Stand at the top of your mat in Mountain pose, big toes touching, heels slightly apart.

Exhale and bend the knees, sending the sitting bones back as if you are sitting in a chair.

Maintain a small gap between the knees.

Make sure you can still see all 10 toes and at least the top half of each foot when you look down.

Raise the arms up over the head, upper arms beside the ears and palms facing each other. (This is challenging so widen the arms if your shoulders are tight.)

Benefits

Chair pose strengthens the thigh muscles, knees and ankles.

It works the abdominal muscles.

Opens the chest.

Chair pose is a total body workout.

Variations

Lift your arms halfway so the hands line up with the shoulders and the palms face down.

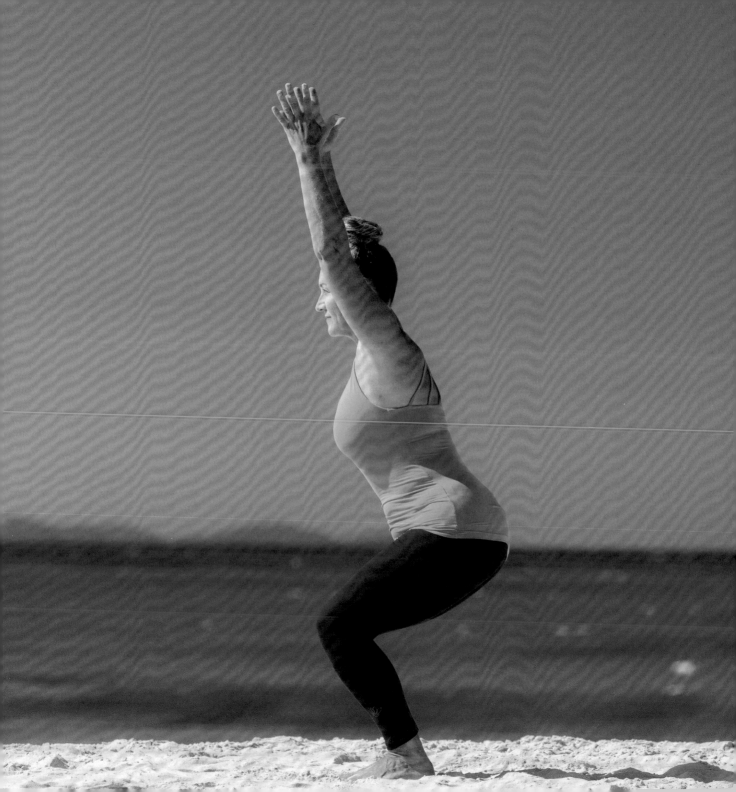

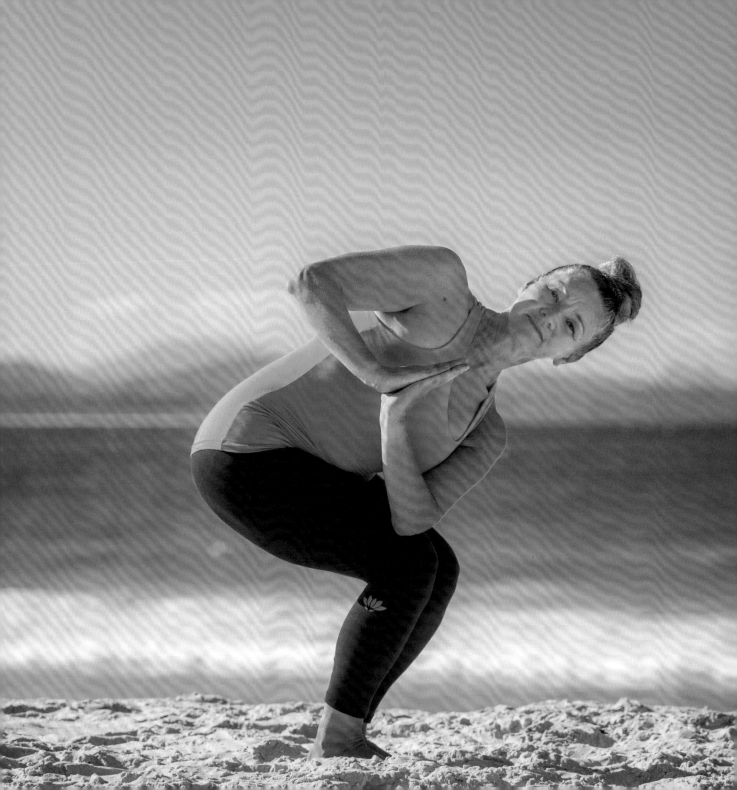

| REVOLVED CHAIR POSE

Come into Chair pose.

Bring your hands into prayer position in the center of the chest.

Turn your torso to the right and hook your upper left arm against your outer right thigh.

Inhale and take the twist deeper.

Exhale, relax and stay in the position.

Look down at your knees and make sure they're level. (This keeps the hips even and protects the lower back.)

Inhale and come back to the chair position keeping the palms pressed together in prayer.

Repeat on the other side.

Exhale and return to Mountain pose.

Benefits

Revolved Chair pose strengthens the thigh muscles, knees and ankles.

It works the abdominal muscles.

Tones the internal organs.

Supports digestion and elimination.

A challenging and heating posture that develops strength and stamina.

Variations

Come into Chair pose and bring the palms into prayer. Turn the torso keeping it upright. Make sure the hips stay facing forward to protect the lower back.

| TRIANGLE POSE

Stand at the top of your mat in Mountain pose, big toes touching, heels slightly apart.

Take a medium step back with your left leg and face towards the left side of your mat.

Line up your right heel with the middle arch of your left foot.

Place your hands on your hips.

Turn your hips slightly so that you face towards your front leg.

Raise the arms to shoulder height and shift the left hip back while deepening the front hip crease.

Feel the hip of the front leg drawing back while the hip of the back leg rolls down to face the floor. (This action helps to release the lower back and increases the length in the underneath side of the torso.)

As the spine lengthens over the front thigh, reach the bottom hand on to the ankle and raise the top arm, lining up the wrist with the shoulder.

Inhale and open the chest more, gazing straight ahead.

Take 5 deep breaths in the posture.

On your next exhalation, ground down into your front foot, inhale and bring the torso upright. Turn both feet to the center.

Repeat on the other side.

BREATHE
STRAIGHTEN
OPEN
INCREASE

Benefits

Triangle pose increases the stretch on the front inner thigh and opens the hamstrings.

It opens the hips.

Increases breath capacity.

Tones the muscles around the kidneys.

Stretches the muscles responsible for side bending.

Works on balance.

Variations

Bend the front knee slightly, if there's tightness along your inner thigh.

Place your front hand on the thigh, if the torso doesn't easily lengthen over your front thigh.

Note that this is not a lateral stretch (side bend). The goal is to have both sides of the torso even. Turning the body to face more towards the front leg will facilitate more length in the upper body, which in turn increases your breath capacity.

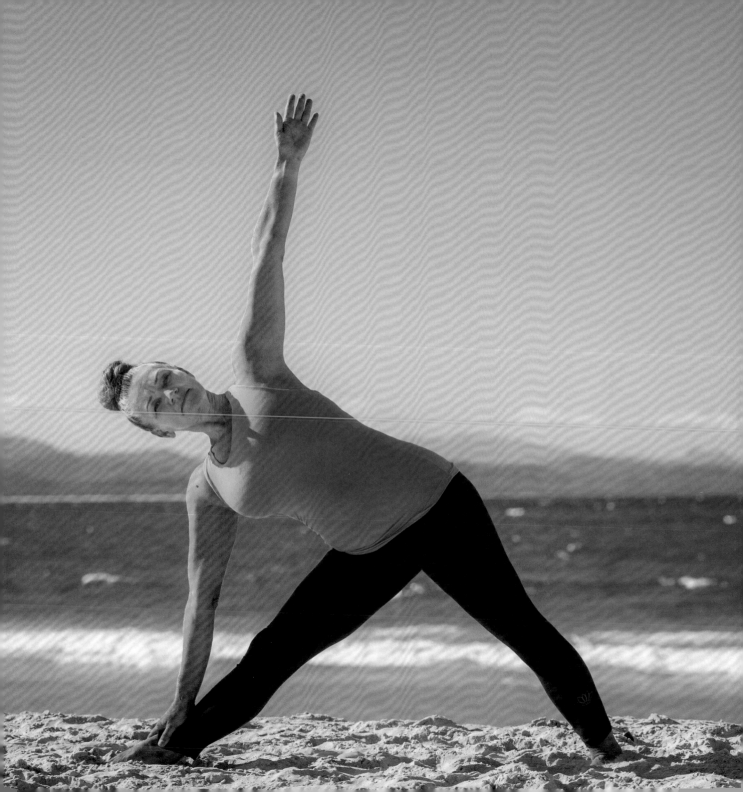

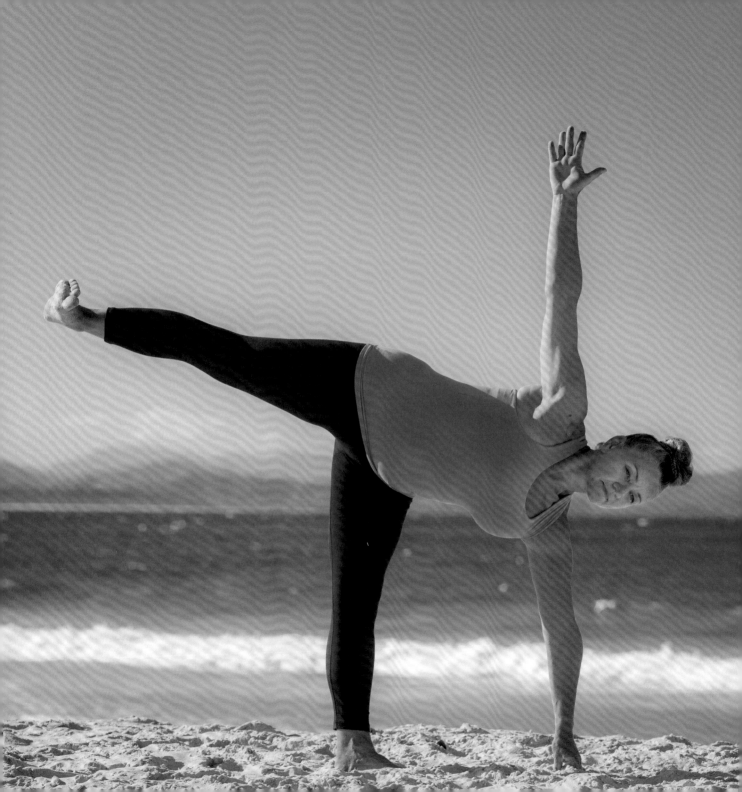

| HALF MOON POSE

Start in Triangle pose on the right side.

Place your right hand on the ground approximately 6 inches in front of your right big toe and place your left hand on your left hip.

Exhale, shifting your weight to your front foot and coming to the left toe tip.

Balancing on your right fingertips, inhale and gently lift your left leg into the air.

Gaze down at your front foot to keep your balance.

The back leg can lift higher than the hip.

Breathe gently in and out working on keeping the balance.

If you feel steady here, raise your left hand into the air keeping the wrist in line with the shoulder.

Exhale and place the lifted leg back down.

Inhale and return to Triangle pose.

Exhale and take a moment to rest.

Inhale and come back to standing, change feet and repeat on the other side.

Benefits

Half Moon pose opens the hips.

It strengthens the ankles, thighs and abdominal muscles.

Develops coordination.

Opens the chest.

Variations

Keep the bottom leg bent and the hand on the hip to balance easily.

Practice this pose with your back against a wall for support.

A good challenge!

| GODDESS POSE

Benefits

Goddess pose builds strength and stamina.

It works the thigh muscles.

Opens the inner thighs.

A heating posture.

Variations

While in the posture, raise your arms, keeping them shoulder-width apart.

Twist to the left as you inhale, hold there, exhale back to center.

Twist to the right as you inhale, hold there, exhale back to center.

If it's challenging to keep your knees over your ankles, tip the pelvis forward. (This also releases the lower back.)

Step the legs wide apart.

Turn the feet out, exhale and bend the knees.

Keep the knees pointed over the toes and lengthen the spine.

Inhale and bring the hands together into prayer position.

Breathe in and out holding the posture until you can feel warmth in the thigh muscles.

On your next inhalation, straighten the legs and stand in Mountain pose at the front of your mat.

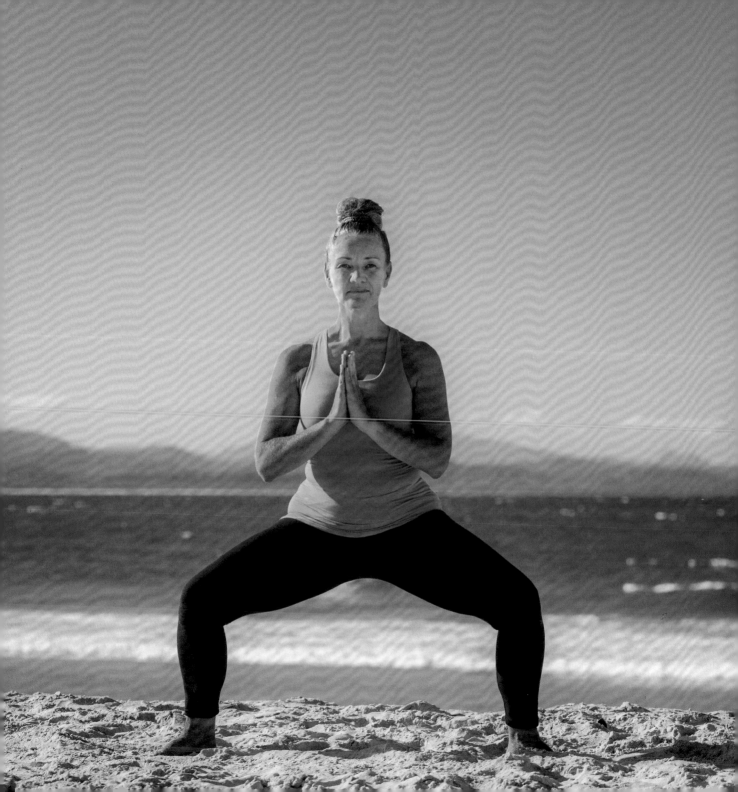

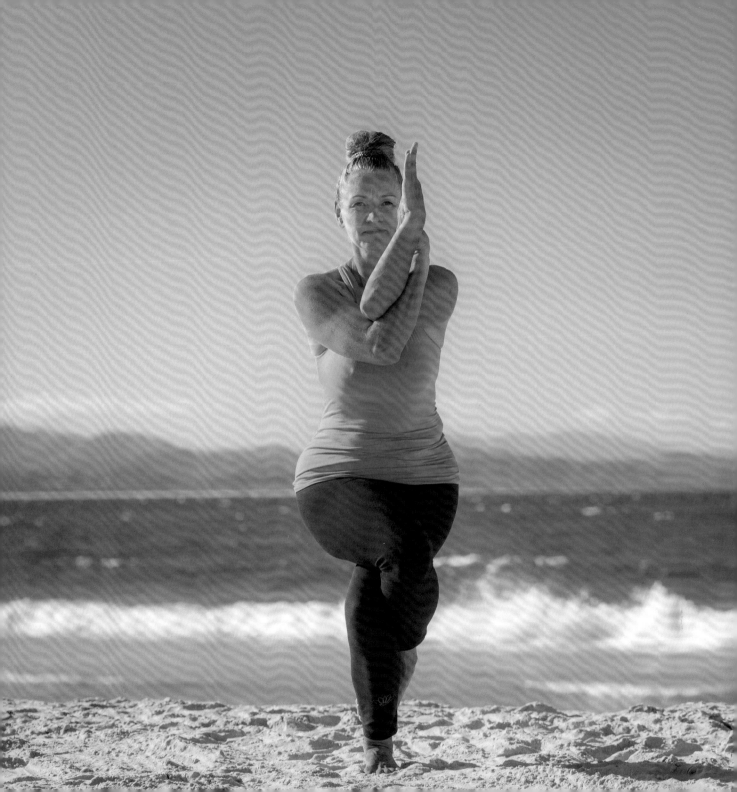

| EAGLE POSE

Come into Mountain pose.

Bend the knees.

Cross your right thigh over your left thigh keeping the ball of the right foot pressed into the ground.

Raise the arms out at shoulder height.

Bend the left elbow and swing your right arm underneath your left upper arm bringing the backs of the palms to touch.

Then bring the palms to touch.

Draw the elbows away from the chest feeling the stretch behind the shoulder blades.

If you feel balanced here, lift the right foot and tuck it behind the right shin.

Breathe gently in and out squeezing the inner thighs and the inner upper arms.

Inhale, extending the arms out the side.

Exhale and return to Mountain pose.

Repeat on the other side.

Benefits

Eagle pose builds heat and develops balance.

It works the inner thighs and strengthens the ankles.

Stretches the deep muscles behind the shoulder blades.

Variations

After crossing the upper arms, take hold of the left wrist with the right hand.

Keep your hands on your hips and just cross the legs.

Stand in Mountain pose and just cross the arms.

| LOCUST POSE

Lie on your belly, forehead pressing into the ground, arms relaxed alongside the body with your thighs, knees and toes all facing down.

Interlace your fingers at the small of your back.

On your next inhalation, lift your feet, legs, upper chest, arms and head off the ground.

Activate the inner thighs and lift them towards the sky while relaxing the buttocks.

Open through the front of the chest, keeping the bottom of your ribs, entire abdomen and pubic bone on the ground.

Keep your neck in line with your spine.

Gaze forwards.

Take 5 to 10 breaths here.

Come down, turn your head to one side and relax.

Benefits

Locust pose works the muscles on either side of the spine, toning the kidneys and adrenals.

It massages the internal organs.

Engages the breath in your upper chest.

Releases the lower back, while working the hamstrings.

Opens the shoulders.

An energizing, stimulating pose.

Variations

Release the hands and have them alongside the body palms facing down.

Extend the arms in front of you palms facing each other. (This is more of a challenge for the upper body.)

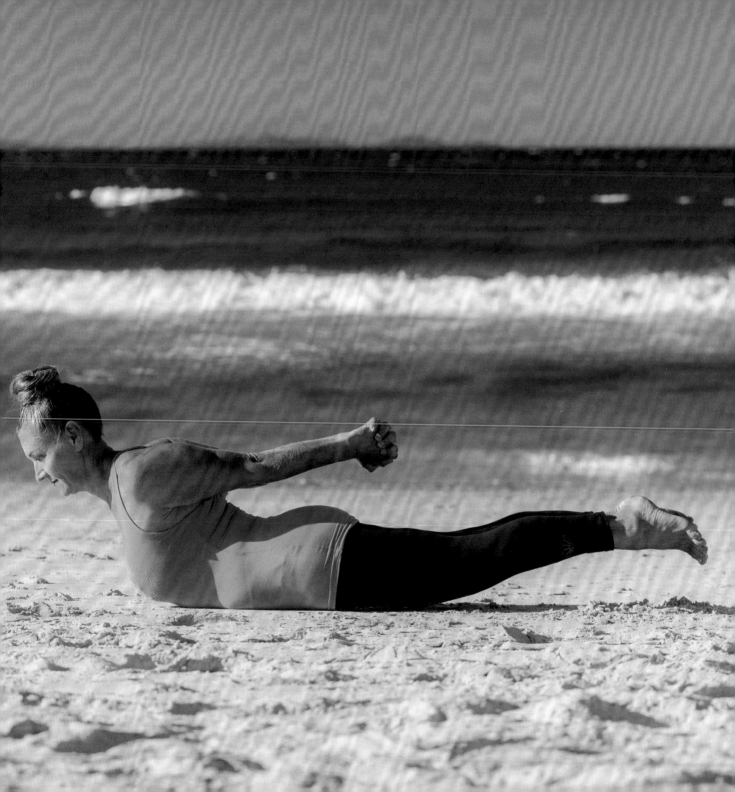

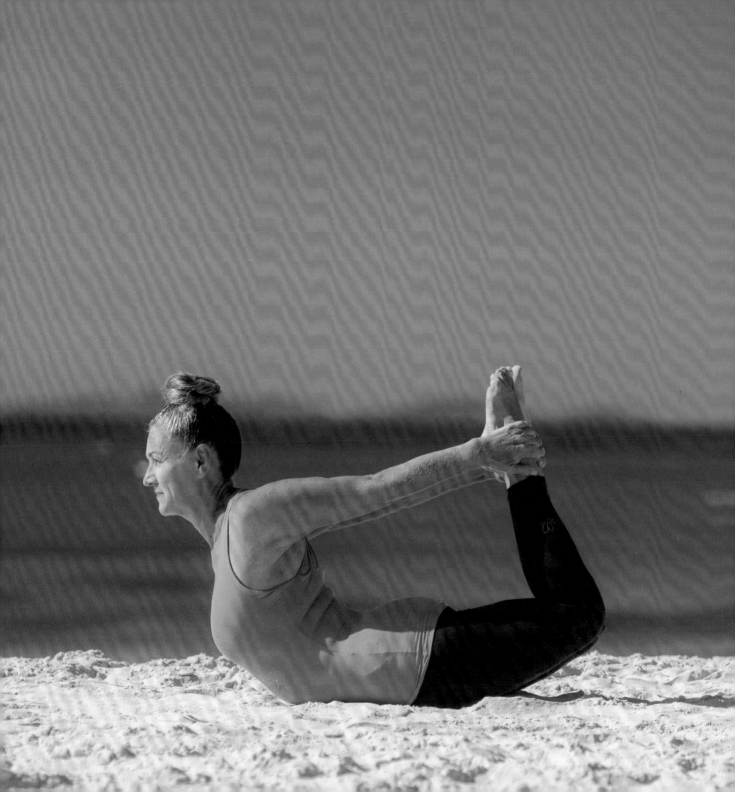

| BOW POSE

INCREASE
DEEPEN
BROADEN
MASSAGE

Lie on your abdomen.

Press your forehead into the ground.

Bend your knees so the heels move towards the buttocks.

Reach back with your hands and grasp your ankles.

Inhale and lift your upper chest, keeping your heels to your buttocks.

If there is no pressure in your lower back or knees, draw the heels away from the buttocks coming into a bow shape.

Breathe deeply into the chest.

Feel the stretch in your shoulders and behind the shoulder blades.

Exhaling, release the posture and lie on your abdomen turning your head to one side.

Repeat the pose.

Benefits

Bow pose provides a deep stretch into the shoulders and upper chest.

It stretches the psoas increasing your breath capacity.

Stretches the thigh muscles.

It's a deep abdominal massage.

Variations

Keep heels to buttocks and isolate the opening in the upper chest.

| CAMEL POSE

Come onto your knees and bring your torso upright.

Place your palms with the fingers pointing towards your waist on your lower back.

Draw the elbows towards each other.

Keeping the length in the neck, inhale, lifting and lengthening the torso and opening the chest.

Maintain a straight line between the hips and the knees.

Exhale and sit the buttocks back to the heels.

Relax in a seated position.

Repeat the pose.

Benefits

Camel opens the chest and the psoas muscle.

It facilitates deep breathing.

Stretches the thigh muscles.

Variation

Place a bolster on your calf muscles and reach your hands back to take hold of the bolster.

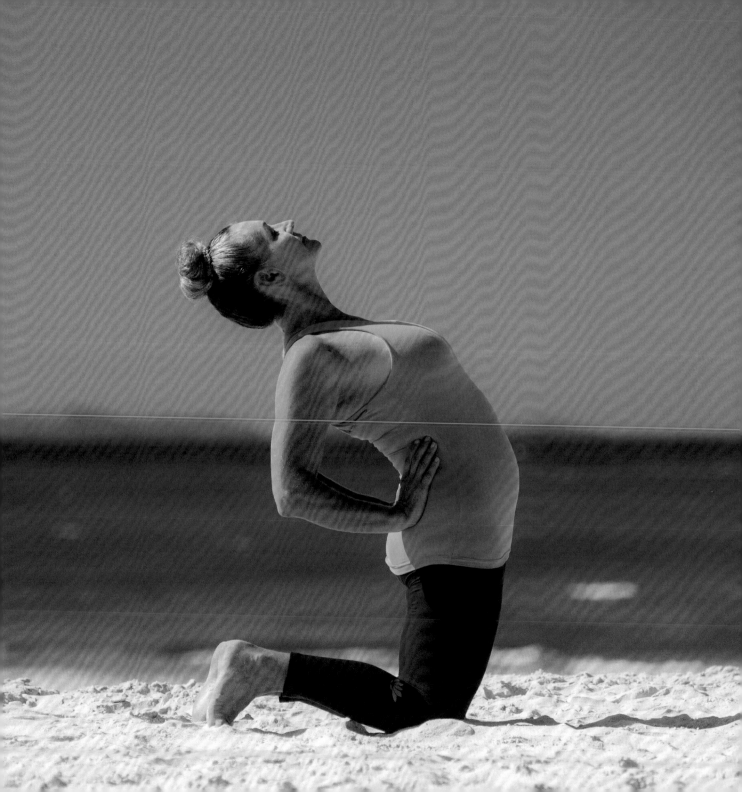

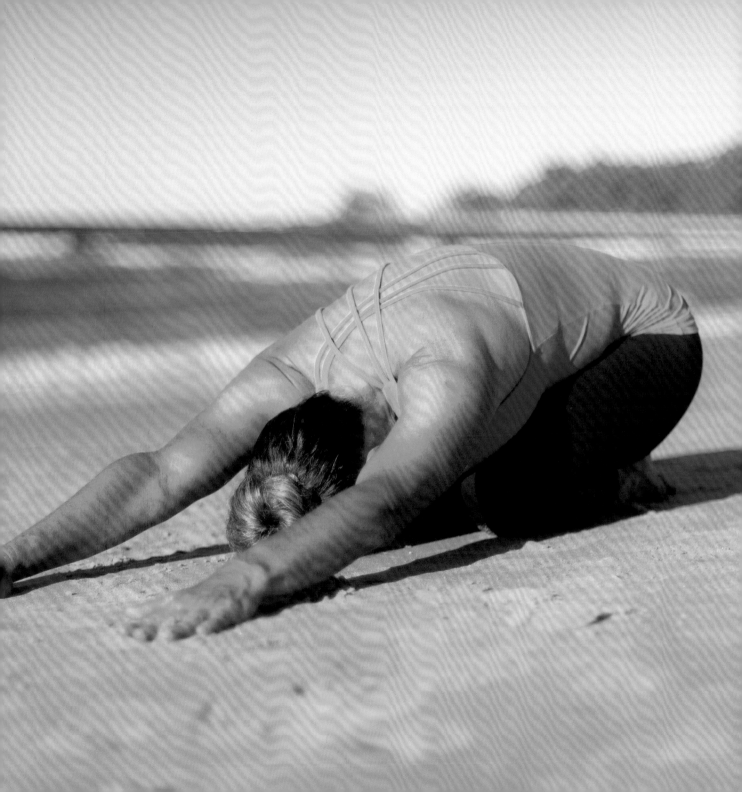

| CHILD POSE

Benefits

Child pose is a neutral position for your spine.

Your head is below your heart, which lowers your blood pressure.

It massages the internal organs.

It's nourishing for the kidneys and adrenals, because the breath is directed towards the back of the body.

A great resting posture.

Variations

Place a block under your forehead, if your head does not easily touch the floor.

Place a bolster behind your knees to create more space, if you are tight in your thighs.

Relax the arms alongside the body to make the pose more passive.

Start on your hands and knees.

Exhaling, send your buttocks back to your heels.

Rest your chest to your thighs, forehead on the ground and have your hands reaching out in front.

Breathe here, feeling the belly pressed against the thighs and the skin on the back of the body stretching.

| BOAT POSE

ENGAGE
TONE
HEAT
BUILD

Sit on your buttocks.

Bend the knees and have the feet flat on the ground and slightly out in front of you.

Place your hands behind your knees, shift the weight back to just behind your sitting bones and come to the tips of your toes.

Lift the feet off the floor keeping the knees bent.

Depending on your balance and strength, you can either have the feet lower than the knees or lift the feet so they line up with the knees.

If you can maintain length in your spine and an open chest, straighten the legs.

Breathe here feeling the core muscles engaged.

Lower the feet back to the ground and place your hands on the ground behind you.

Benefits

Boat pose strengthens the core.

It builds heat.

Tones the abdominals.

Engages the thigh muscles.

An effective counter pose to the back bends.

Variations

Keep the knees bent.

Hold on behind your knees and straighten the legs to help you balance.

Take hold of both big toes with your index and middle fingers and straighten the legs. (This one is very challenging.)

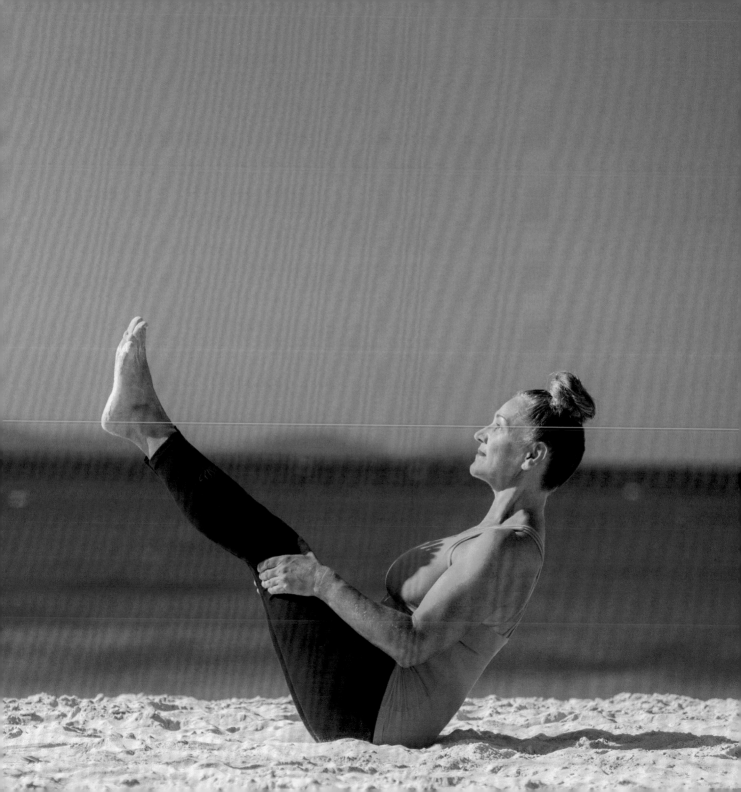

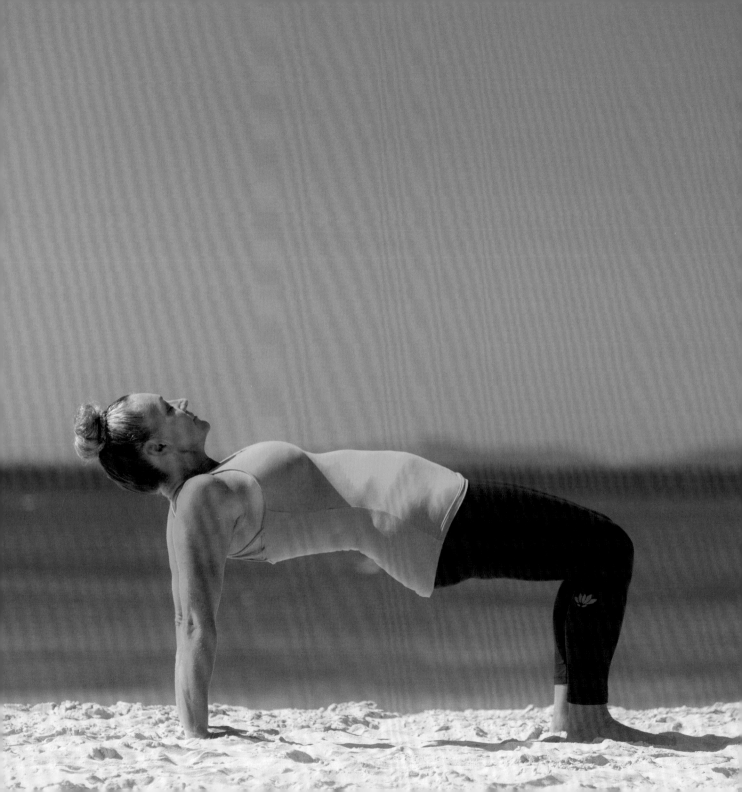

| TABLE POSE

Bend the knees and have the feet flat on the ground slightly out in front of your knees.

Place the hands on the ground behind you, fingers pointing towards the buttocks.

Inhale and lift the pelvis towards the sky as you keep the chin in towards your chest.

The knees and ankles are in line with the feet, inner-hip-width apart.

Breathe deeply.

Exhale, lowering the pelvis.

Return to the starting position.

Repeat the pose.

Benefits

Table pose opens the chest and releases the shoulder blades.

It stretches the abdominals.

Strengthens the wrists.

A challenging and heating posture.

Variations

Turn the hands to face away from the buttocks and move into the posture.

Balance on your fists if the wrists hurt.

Keep the hips closer to the floor only lifting the pelvis halfway.

| HEAD TO KNEE POSE

OPEN
NURTURE
LENGTHEN
ELONGATE

Sit on your buttocks with both legs extended out in front of you.

Bend the right knee and place the sole of the foot close to the groin on the inside of the left thigh.

Flex both feet, activating the extended leg, while keeping the knee facing towards the sky.

Inhaling, lengthen the spine and begin to fold forward from the hips.

Exhaling, reach the hands to either side of the leg.

Only take hold of the foot if your abdomen easily touches your thigh.

Most importantly, keep the chest open and breathe deeply.

On your next inhalation, return to the upright position and repeat the posture on the other side.

Benefits

Head to Knee pose is a great stretch for the hamstrings.

It opens the hips.

Stretches and tones the adrenals and kidneys.

A calming and relaxing posture.

Variation

Bend the knee of the extended leg, if you feel a pulling on your lower back or in your hamstrings. Rest your abdomen on your thigh. (See modifications p.296)

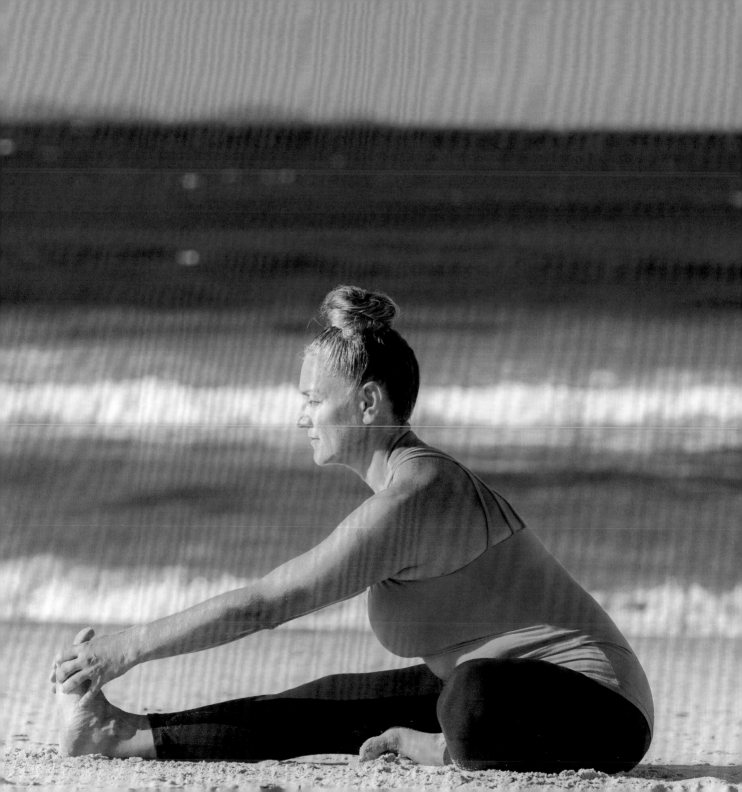

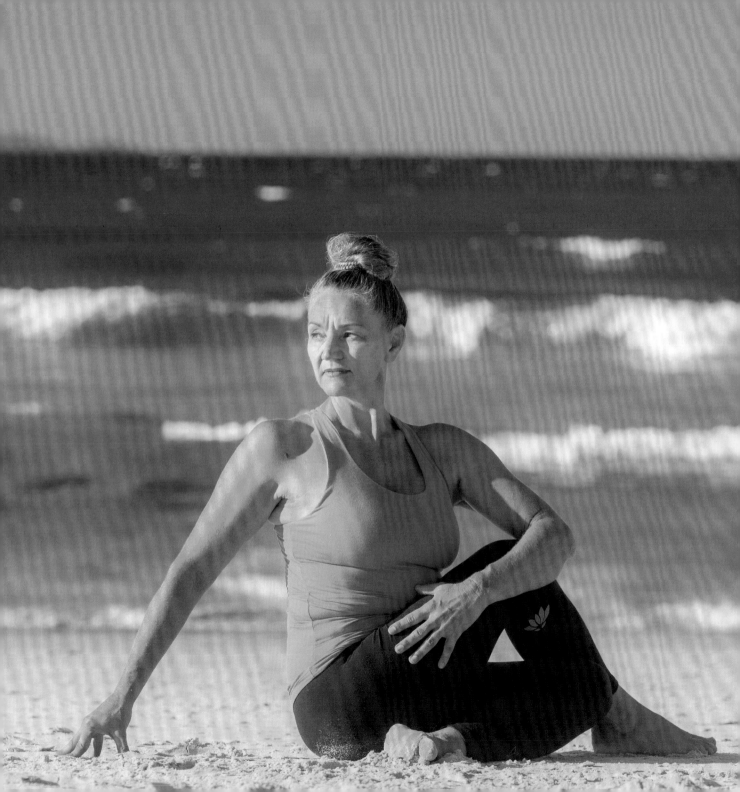

| HALF SEATED SPINAL TWIST

REFRESH
NOURISH
DETOXIFY
TONE

Sit on your buttocks with both legs extended out in front of you.

Bend you right knee and cross your right foot over your left leg. (The right foot is facing the same direction as your extended leg and is flat on the ground.)

Bend your left knee and place the heel of your left foot beside the outer right hip.

Place your right hand on the ground behind you, the heel of your hand in line with the center of your spine and slightly away from the body.

Inhale and extend your left arm high into the air, then twist the upper body to the right, wrapping your upper left arm around your outer right thigh.

Exhale and relax.

Inhale and twist further making sure the movement for the twist is coming from the torso and not the head.

Gaze in the direction you are twisting.

Breathe deeply.

Turn back to center, unwind the legs and repeat the posture on the other side.

Benefits

Half Seated Spinal Twist is a deep spinal twist that forces the breath into areas it wouldn't normally reach.

It's a massage for the ascending and descending colon.

It brings fresh blood into the spine.

It's nourishing for the internal organs.

It is an outer hip opener.

Variation

If the hips are tight, keep the left leg straight.

Bring the upper left arm to the outside of the right thigh to deepen the twist.

| CORPSE POSE

REPLENISH
HEAL
RELAX
SURRENDER

Lie on your back.

Have your arms and legs slightly away from the body, palms facing upwards, feet relaxed and open.

Turn the head gently from side to side until it rests in the center.

If your chin juts up towards the sky, place a blanket underneath your head.

Relax completely.

Don't worry about the breath or what the body is doing.

Feel how effortless it is to lie here.

Stay here for at least 5 minutes.

When you are ready, roll to one side and come up.

Benefits

This is the most important posture in the sequence. Missing this posture is like making a meal and then deciding not to eat it.

All the nourishing and healing benefits of the practice are integrated in this posture.

The relaxed part of the nervous system is engaged.

The body releases and relaxes at a cellular level.

The glandular system is replenished.

The alpha and theta brainwaves are dominant and the mind relaxes.

Variation

Place a bolster under your knees, if there is pressure in your lower back.

Place an inch-thick folded blanket under the head, if there is any tension in the neck.

Place an eye pillow over your eyes, if you have an active mind.

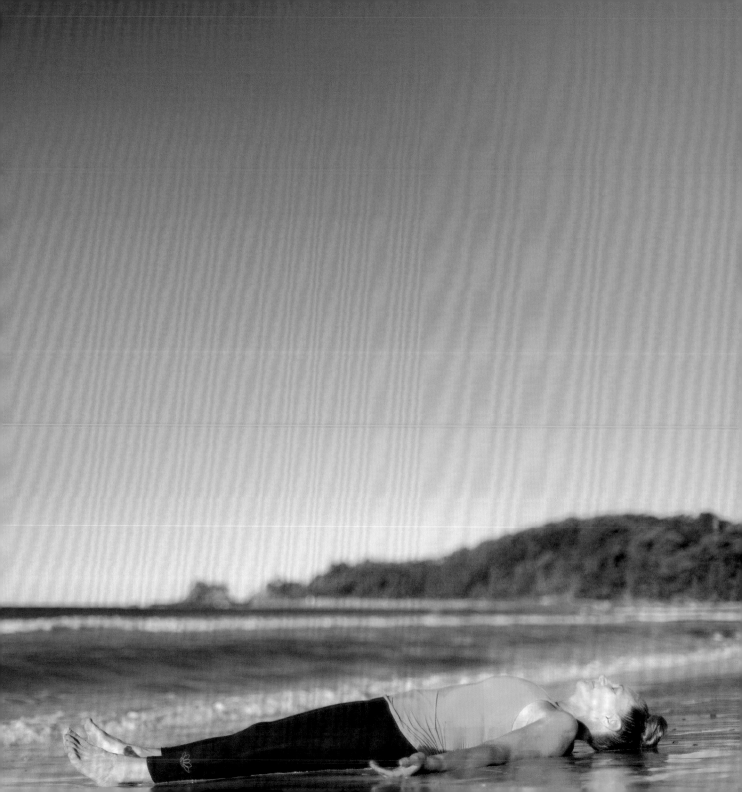

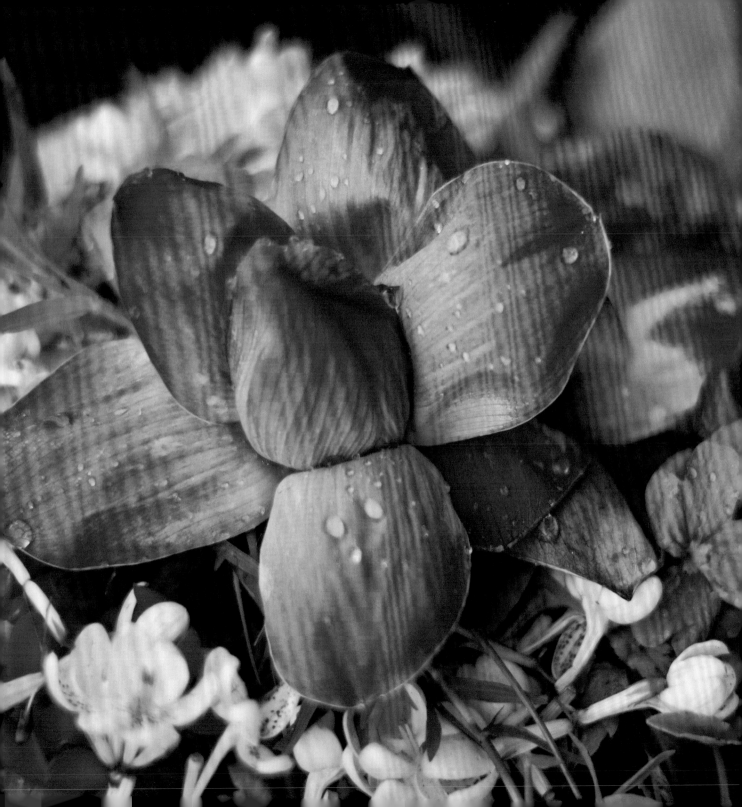

I YOGA NIDRA

I recommend recording the yoga nidra so that you can take yourself
through the practice anytime you feel the need to take a longer rest.

Getting settled

Lie flat on your back and completely let go.
Feel how gravity holds the body on the mat.
You don't have to do a thing.
Give your body up to the force of gravity.
Feel how gravity, like a huge magnet, draws the body into the earth.
Feel how the earth supports the body. Unconditionally.
Let go of all effort.
Let go of the need to do anything.
Let go of the need to let go.
Everything is going on absolutely effortlessly.
The whole of creation is going on without effort.
Feel the breath moving through your nose.
Feel your heart beat.
Feel how effortless it is.
Feel the coolness in the breath as it moves through each nostril.

Relaxation of the different body parts

Bring your awareness into your feet and feel where the heels touch the floor.
Feel those two points relaxing.
Feel where the calf muscles touch the floor.
Feel those two points relax completely.
Moving up to the thighs, feel where the thighs touch the floor.
Feel those two points relax completely.
Feel where the buttocks touch the floor.
Moving into the lower back, feel it relax completely.
The upper back relaxing.
Feel where the shoulders touch the floor relaxing.
Moving into the belly, feel all tension letting go.
All tension drains from the belly into the earth.
As you let it go, it lets you go.
Feel the neck muscles relaxing.
Shoulders relaxing.
Feel the arms relaxing.
Feel where the elbows touch the floor, forearms touch the floor.
Feel where the hands touch the floor.
Feel those two points relaxing.

Color visualization

Bring all your awareness into the back of your head, where the back of the head touches the floor.
Feel that point at the very top of the spine, the base of the skull.
Feel a blue light emerging from that point, the color of the sky.
Feel this electric blue light washing through the whole top of the head.
In the very center of the brain, feel a golden egg resting there, emitting a golden liquid light.
Feel this gold liquid light emerging through the top of your head washing forward towards the forehead where it trickles down.
The golden liquid light relaxes the eyes.
Feel the eyes dropping into the back of the head into the pools of golden light, washing through the cheeks, nose, lips and jaw.
Your tongue lulls into the back of the throat as your relax completely.
The whole body is without tension.
Each muscle and each joint completely relaxed.

Rest here for 5 more minutes.

Coming back to normal waking consciousness.

Now feeling the breath again through the nose.
Bring your awareness back to the heart and feel your heart beating.
Try to pick up your heartbeat.
Feeling the coolness of the breath in your nostrils.
Gently wiggle your fingers and your toes.
Stretching your arms up over your head.
Gently roll to one side and stay there for a few moments.
When you are ready, come up to a comfortable seated position.
Bring your palms to rest at your heart, bow your head and take a moment for yourself.

Namaste.

| APPENDIX A

If you've landed on this page, it means you want to find easier versions of some of the postures in your sequence. I like to modify postures when I'm tired, feeling a bit tighter or having trouble balancing. Some days I don't have as much strength either, especially if my blood sugar is higher or lower.

Some people think modifying a pose is a cop out, but let me reassure you. When you modify, you are honoring yourself, your body and its fluctuating rhythms. I find that when I start a practice with modifications I open up slowly and safely. It doesn't take much time before I can do the pose in the sequence again.

| Modifications

Rather than sharing a modification for every pose in the sequence, I've chosen the ones that I feel are supportive and easy to do.

Use the color-coded key pictured below, to select the appropriate modification for each sequence.

● VATA SEQUENCE

● PITTA SEQUENCE

● KAPHA SEQUENCE

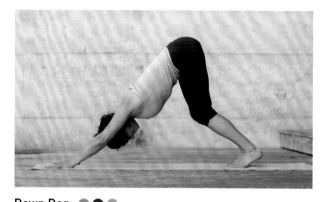

Down Dog ●●●
Bend your knees, if your hamstrings are tight or you feel a pulling on your lower back.

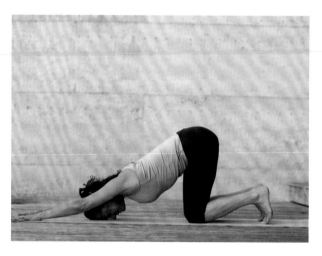

Half Dog Pose ●●●
Come into half dog, if you have pain in your wrists or weak arms. Rest on your knees and walk your hands as far forward as possible so your torso is extended and the spine is lengthened. Breathe deeply, feeling the stretch in the armpits.

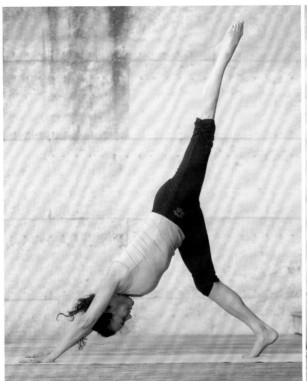 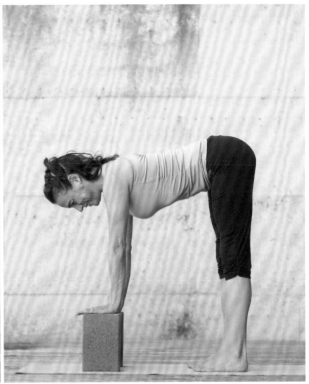

One Point Pose ●

Bend the standing leg knee, if the hamstring is tight.

Full Forward Fold ● ●

Straighten your legs and place your hands on blocks directly under your shoulders, bringing the ground to you, if it hurts more in your lower back when you bend the knees in the posture. Bring the spine into a flat back, crown of the head in line with the tailbone.

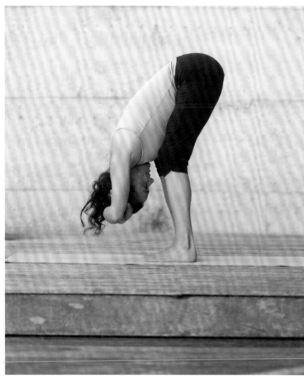

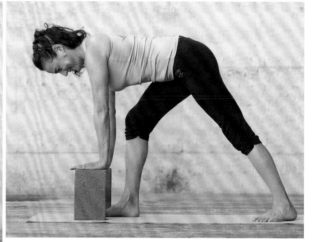

Triangle Forward Bend ● ●
Place the hands on blocks underneath the
shoulders and bend the front knee, if the front
hamstring is tight.

Full Forward Fold - Modification 2 ●
Start in Down Dog. Walk your feet to your hands.
Bend your knees so that your belly rests on your
thighs.

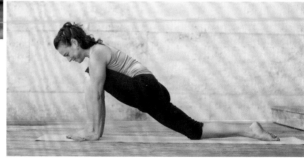

Low Lunge ● ●
Keep the torso relaxed over the front thigh, hands on
either side of the front foot.

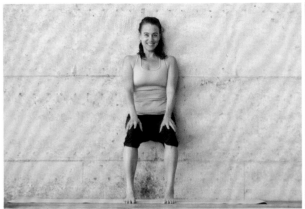

Chair pose ●

Take your buttocks back to a wall for extra support.

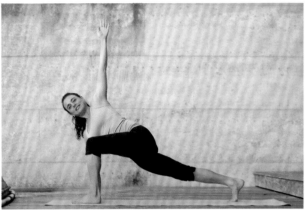

Revolved Right Angle ●

Place the right hand under the right shoulder and raise the left arm, keeping left wrist and left shoulder stacked.

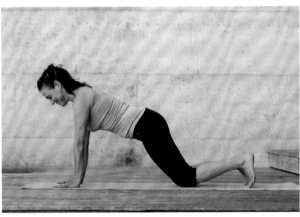

Plank pose ●

Rest on the knees, bringing slightly more weight into the wrists to work the upper body.

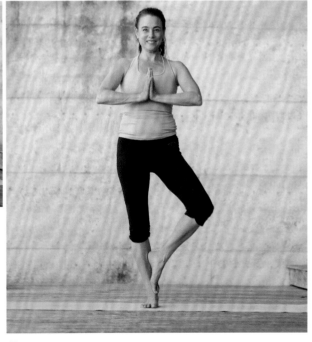

Tree pose ●

Place the left foot along the inside of the right shin.

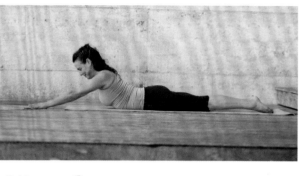

Sphinx pose ●

Walk the hands further away, lift the elbows while straightening the arms, if there is strain in the lower back.

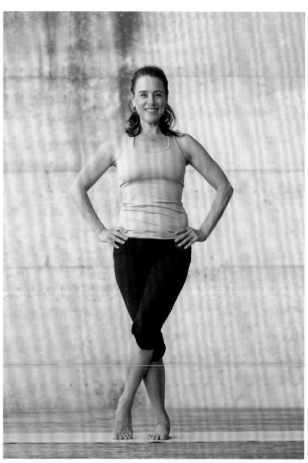

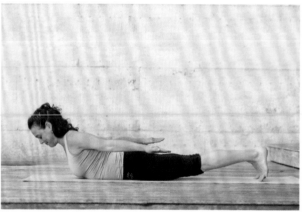
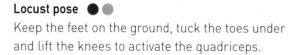

Eagle pose ●

When you cross the thighs, keep the ball of the foot on the floor and deeply bend the knees.

Locust pose ● ●

Keep the feet on the ground, tuck the toes under and lift the knees to activate the quadriceps.

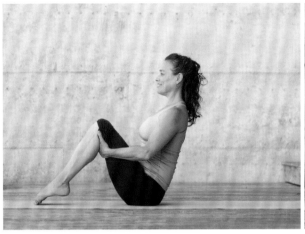

Boat pose ●●

Keep toes on the floor, holding behind the knees. Maintain a long spine and open chest.

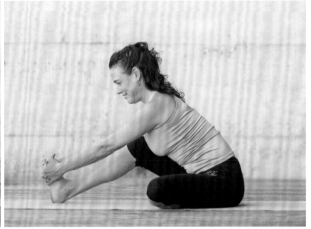

Head to Knee pose ●●

Bend the knee of the extended leg, if you feel a pulling on your lower back or in your hamstrings and rest your abdomen on your thigh.

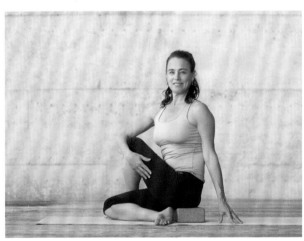

Half Seated Spinal Twist pose ●

If the hips are tight, keep the left leg straight. Sit on a blanket or block, if you tend to sit more to the back of your sitting bones.

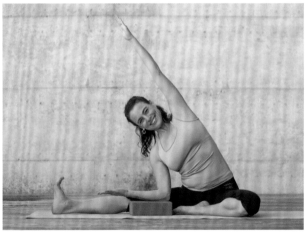

Revolved Head to Knee pose ●

Rest your lower arm on a block bringing the ground to you. Reach your arm alongside your ear.

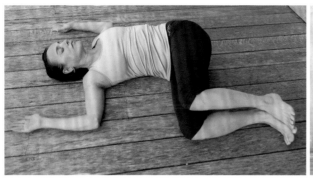

Maltese Twist pose ●
Bend the arms at the elbows.

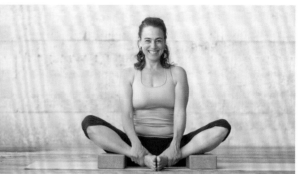

Cobbler pose ●
For more comfort in the pose, place blocks underneath the thighs.

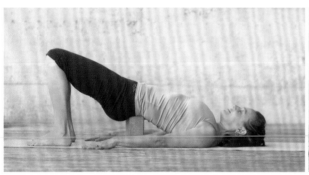

Bridge pose ●
Rest your lower back on a block, if there is strain in the knees. A good modification if the posture hurts your lower back or you have neck issues.

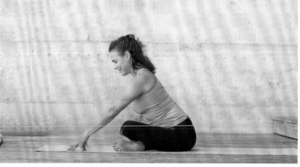

Easy Cross-Legged Seat ●
Keep your spine upright and place your hands just a few inches in front to maintain length in your spine.

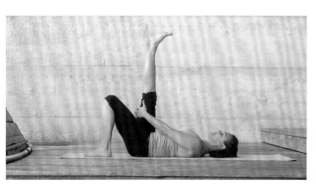

Resting Extended Leg pose ●
Bend the knee of the leg along the ground, if there is any pain or tightness in the lower back.

| PSOAS SEQUENCE

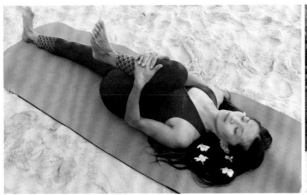

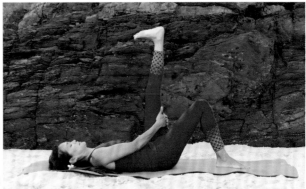

Wind Expeller Pose

Lie on your back with the legs extended and parallel to each other.

Feel your length from the crown of your head to your tailbone.

Bend the right knee and interlace the fingers over the shin.

Gently draw the thigh towards your chest.

Keep your heel in line with your knee.

Flex evenly through both feet, activating the legs.

Draw the tailbone down to the floor, feeling the lower back lengthening along the floor.

As you breathe in and out, feel the right side of your belly receiving a deep massage.

Hold here for 5 to 10 breaths.

Release the leg and repeat on the other side.

Resting Extended Leg Pose Variation 1

Lie on your back with the legs extended and parallel to each other.

Feel length from the crown of your head to your tailbone.

Bend the right knee and interlace the fingers behind the thigh.

Bend the knee of the leg along the ground,

Extend the foot to the sky keeping the leg straight and the thigh muscle engaged.

Press the back of your thigh into your hands and your hands into your thigh creating a feeling of resistance. (This will co-activate the muscles around the thigh bone and increase the effectiveness of the stretch.)

Breathe deeply into the chest.

Hold here for 5 to 10 breaths.

Release the leg and repeat on the other side.

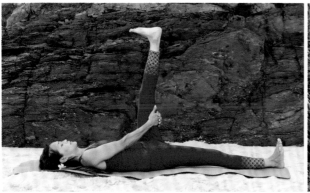 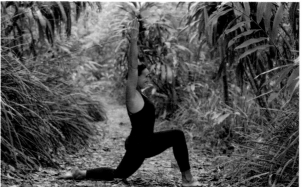

Resting Extended Leg Pose Variation 2

Lie on your back with the legs extended and parallel to each other.

Feel length from the crown of your head to your tailbone.

Bend the right knee and interlace the fingers behind the thigh.

Extend the foot to the sky keeping the leg straight and the thigh muscle engaged.

Press the back of your thigh into your hands and your hands into your thigh creating a feeling of resistance. (This will co-activate the muscles around the thigh bone and increase the effectiveness of the stretch.)

Make sure the leg along the ground is straight with the knee facing towards the sky.

Flex both feet.

Breathe deeply into the chest.

Hold here for 5 to 10 breaths.

Release the leg and repeat on the other side.

Low Lunge pose

Start in Down Dog pose.

Step your right foot far enough forward in between your hands so that the heel of your front foot is lined up with the heels of both hands.

Bring your torso into an upright position, keeping your hands on your hips.

Check to make sure your knee is directly over your ankle in a stacked position.

Raise your arms into the air and keep the arms shoulder width apart.

Keep the shoulders relaxed and gaze straight ahead.

Deepen the bend in the knee to feel the stretch in the hip flexor of the left leg.

Open the chest and breathe deeply.

Hold here for 5 to 10 breaths.

Bring the hands back down to either side of the right foot and step back into Down Dog.

Repeat on the other side.

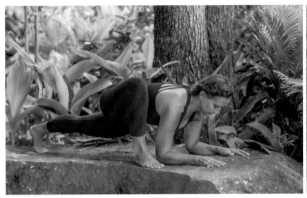 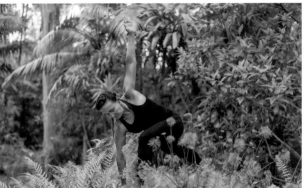

Lizard Pose

Start in Down Dog pose.

Step your right foot far enough forward in between your hands so that the heel of your front foot is lined up with the heels of both hands.

Turn your right foot slightly out to the side and place both hands on the inside of your right foot, then lower onto your forearms.

Keep the spine extended, feeling the length from your tailbone to your crown.

Squeeze your inner right thigh, pressing it against the right side of the torso.

Extend the back of your neck.

Feel the stretch in the front of the left groin.

Hold here for 5 to 10 breaths.

Step back into Down Dog.

Repeat on the other side.

Revolved Right Angle Pose

Come onto your hands and knees.

Step your left foot in between your hands

Check to make sure your front knee is stacked over your ankle and that your back hip and back knee are in line.

As you move into the pose, your hip will come slightly forward out of alignment.

Place the right hand under the right shoulder and raise the left arm, keeping left wrist and left shoulder stacked.

Lift your right knee off the floor and straighten your back leg.

Take 5 deep breaths here twisting deeper on the inhalation and resting in place on the exhalation.

Bring your left hand back down to the floor on your final exhalation.

Return to your hands and knees and repeat on the other side.

| Symptoms and Remedies at a Glance

In case you're curious to know more about how specific postures, practices and yoga sequences can benefit the varied symptoms associated with diabetes I've put together a chart with symptoms and remedies at a glance.

What I've discovered through my own explorations and years of study is that a yoga practice for diabetes is not 'one size fits all'. Yoga is not a pill we can take. If it were, I would be cured!

However, knowing your constitution and the poses and practices specific to that constitution will support you in achieving better overall health and wellbeing as you navigate a life with diabetes.

In the following chart I have grouped similar symptoms together and listed the associated practices and postures that can be performed either separately or together to help manage those symptoms

Diabetes is unpredictable, the body is changeable as are the external factors that affect our day to day lives. Keep in mind that consistency of practice will garner results. Once you're ready to tackle a symptom stick with the recommended pose, practice or sequence for at least six weeks, consider keeping a diary so you can track your results. Be curious. You might even discover that other symptoms in other categories will also benefit from the practice you have chosen to explore.

Once you've experienced the practice for yourself and discovered (according to the needs of your type) how motivating, calming and restorative yoga can be I'm confident that the results will speak for themselves.

DIABETES SYMPTOMS	AYURVEDIC DOSHA IT RELATES TO	BENEFICIAL YOGA SEQUENCES (chapter 7)	
sleep issues, insomnia, anxiety, fear	vata and pitta	vata balancing pitta balancing	
sedentary lifestyle, lethargy due to high blood sugars, lack of energy, weight gain, obesity, cravings, visceral and abdominal fat, depression	kapha and pitta	kapha balancing pitta balancing	
diabetes burnout, diabulimia, overwhelm of managing a chronic disease, poor self image, shame and guilt	vata, pitta, kapha	vata balancing pitta balancing kapha balancing	
insulin resistance, poor cardiovascular or vascular systems, circulation, neuropathy	kapha, vata	kapha balancing vata balancing	
digestive issues, gastroparesis, bowel function—constipation	vata, pitta, kapha	vata balancing pitta balancing kapha balancing	
kidney issues, nephropathy, bladder infections, adrenal fatigue, multiple autoimmune diseases, retinopathy, gum disease, hearing loss, heart disease	vata	vata balancing/pitta balancing with a very gentle approach	

BREATHING PRACTICE CONCENTRATION PRACTICE DAILY ROUTINE	SPECIFIC POSTURES THAT ARE OF BENEFIT (You can do one posture on its own and hold for 10 breaths or practice all the postures as a sequence.)
full complete breath, ocean breath, sunrise meditation, soham meditation, yoga nidra, sesame oil on feet and head	child pose, easy cross-legged seat, down dog, full forward fold, fan, triangle forward bend, child pose variation, bridge, wind expeller, resting extended leg, maltese twist, head to knee, wide angle seated, cobbler, cow face, inverted leg, reclining buddha, corpse
ocean breath, walk in the early morning or after dinner, satyam meditation	moving cat, tiger, plank, down dog, one point, low lunge, lizard, warrior 2, crescent, goddess, chair, revolved chair, revolved right angle, boat, sphinx, baby cobra, locust, bow, camel, bridge, table, sage, half seated spinal twist, easy cross-legged seat
full complete breath, alternate nostril breath, sunrise meditation, satyam meditation, sesame oil on feet and head, yoga nidra	moving cat, tiger, plank, down dog, one point, prepare, full forward fold, mountain, moon, warrior 2, triangle, half moon, fan, eagle, tree, baby cobra, locust, bow, child pose variation, cobblers, easy cross-legged seat, corpse
satyam meditation, sesame oil on feet and head, walk in the early morning or after dinner	moving cat, tiger, plank, down dog, one point, low lunge, prepare, warrior 2, crescent, triangle, goddess, chair, revolved chair, moon, eagle, revolved right angle, boat, locust, bow, child pose variation, sage, half seated spinal twist, revolved head to knee, head to knee, wide angle seated, cobbler, inverted leg, reclining buddha
full complete breath, sunrise meditation, yoga nidra	child pose, full forward fold, low lunge, lizard, triangle, forward bend, moon, revolved chair, sphinx, baby cobra, locust pose, bow, child pose variation, sage, half seated spinal twist, revolved head to knee, head to knee, wind expeller, maltese twist, corpse
full complete breath, ocean breath, sunrise meditation, soham meditation, yoga nidra	child pose, child pose variation, easy cross-legged seat, Half dog (p. 291), low lunge (p. 293), head to knee (p. 296), supported bridge (p. 297), wind expeller, maltese twist, inverted leg, reclining buddha, corpse

| Yoga Resources

Divine Goddess Yoga Products

Heartfelt yoga clothing and products designed with practice and love in mind. We specialize in eco-friendly, biodegradable yoga mats and natural fiber yoga clothing. We believe that the practice of yoga has the power to change lives and create love.

www.divinegoddess.net

Yoga Trail

YogaTrail is the yoga network where yogis connect with their teachers and studios. Great for finding your yoga, but even better for keeping up with what's happening in your own yoga world - around town and around the globe.

www.yogatrail.com

YogaMate.org

A digital platform for the global yogic community - helping spread awareness around the depth, breadth and healing applications of yoga. Find, connect with and be inspired on your path to wellbeing.

www.YogaMate.org

Yoga Mats and Props online

www.empind.com.au

| Ayurveda Recommended Reading

Ayurveda: The science of self-healing, Dr. Vasant Lad

Yoga and Ayurveda: Self-Healing and Self-Realization, Dr. David Frawley

Prakruti: Your Ayurvedic Constitution, Robert E. Svoboda

The Complete Book of Ayurvedic Home Remedies, Dr. Vasant Lad

The Path of Practice, Maya Tiwari

Ayurvedic Healing for Women, Atreya

The Ayurvedic Cook Book: A Personalized Guide to Good Nutrition and Health, Amadea Morningstar and Urmila Desai

| Diabetes Resources

Diabetes Dominator

Daniele Hargenrader is a bestselling author, nutritionist, health coach, international speaker, and certified personal trainer. She helps individuals from all walks of life to think, eat, and move in ways that allow them to achieve a quality of health and life they previously thought unattainable through our powers of choice and self-love.

www.diabetesdominator.com

Dr. Jody Stanislaw, naturopathic doctor, certified diabetes educator

Dr. Jody Stanislaw works with people with type 1 diabetes located anywhere around the globe via phone/Skype. Being a type 1 herself plus a holistic physician, patients receive help from a holistic perspective, which includes nutrition, fitness, and emotional support, as well as getting their diabetes under excellent control.

www.DrJodyND.com

www.consultwithdrjody.com/type1 to sign up for a complimentary intro consult

www.consultwithdrjody.com/groupprogram to sign up for her monthly diabetes group program

Beyond Type 1

Beyond Type 1 seeks to bring a new level of respect, understanding and support for those living with type 1 diabetes. Our goal is to highlight the brilliance of those fighting this disease every day and provide important resources for those living with and affected by type 1 while always working toward ensuring a cure is on its way.

www.beyondtype1.org

Diabetes Daily

Helping people with type 1 and type 2 diabetes live a better life!

www.diabetesdaily.com

Insulin Nation

Insulin Nation is a website that provides news, insight and opinion on diabetes treatment and life with type 1 diabetes.

www.insulinnation.com

Diabetics Doing Things

Diabetics Doing Things exists to tell the inspiring stories of type 1 diabetics around the world, in hopes of bringing hope, inspiration and education to those who need it.

www.diabeticsdoingthings.com

Diabetes Daily Grind & Real Life Diabetes Podcast

Real support for the diabetes life. Help us inspire people with the disease to be brave as they live out their authentic type 1 and type 2 diabetes lives!

www.diabetesdailygrind.com

We Are Diabetes

We Are Diabetes is an organization primarily devoted to promoting support and awareness for type 1 diabetics who suffer from eating disorders. WAD is dedicated to providing guidance, hope and resources to those who may be struggling, as well as to their families and loved ones.

www.wearediabetes.org

Delphi Diabetes Coaching

Know Yourself, Know Your Diabetes

Leann offers emotional strength and a supportive environment for people with diabetes. She works with your feelings and thoughts and help you thrive - not just survive - with diabetes. She doesn't believe in a one-size-fits-all view of diabetes management and works with you wherever you are to determine what's important to you and what really helps you take care of yourself.

www.DelphiDiabetesCoaching.com

Diabetes Alive Incorporated

Diabetes Alive offers type 1 diabetics assistance through raising money for research providing information and support through mental health counseling, advocacy and specialized products. We also support type 2 diabetics in mental health and nutritional support.

www.diabetesalive.org.au

Diabetes Connections

A weekly podcast sharing stories of connection to educate and inspire. Hosted by long-time broadcaster and diabetes mom Stacey Simms.

www.diabetes-connections.com

THE BETES Organization, Inc.

Health Care is a Human Story

THE BETES mission is to pave a path to joyful health for all people who carry chronic health conditions through unique creative programming.

www.thebetes.org

Beta Cell

Beta Cell is a podcast about the people living with type 1 diabetes.

www.betacellpodcast.com

A Sweet Life

The diabetes magazine by people with diabetes for people with diabetes.

www.asweetlife.org

Cynthia Zuber - Diabetes Light: My holistic journey to health

Cynthia has lived with type 1 diabetes for 29 years and also lives with other autoimmune conditions including hypothyroidism and food sensitivities. She uses a holistic, nutritional and lifestyle approach to feel her best in body, mind and spirit. She loves sharing her journey to help others.

www.diabeteslight.com

| Pose Index

I ABOUT THE AUTHOR

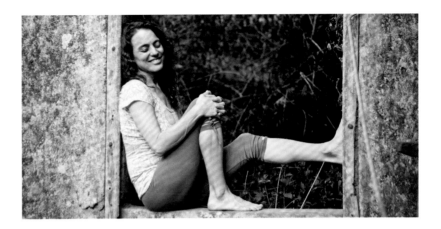

Rachel Zinman was diagnosed with diabetes in 2008. It took six years for her to accept her diagnosis of type 1 LADA diabetes. She started yoga in high school when she was 17 and by the age of 19 she was hooked.

Rachel is passionate about the deeper aspects of yoga and its ability to heal and inspire. She has spent the last 30 years practicing passionately as well as teaching nationally (in Australia) and internationally since 1992.

Rachel is a published poet and author, award-winning musician, mother, partner and amateur film maker. She started her Yoga For Diabetes blog to share with the diabetes online community how yoga has helped her manage diabetes.

Rachel's articles on yoga and diabetes have been featured in Elephant Journal, Diabetes Daily, A Sweet Life, Insulin Nation, Beyond Type 1, Diabetes Counselling Online, Diabetes Alive, Veranda Magazine, Yoga Trail, Yoga4tv, Mind Body Green and DoYouYoga and most recently in the #1 bestseller, Unleash Your Inner Diabetes Dominator. She is a featured expert for several online resources for yoga and diabetes.

You can find out more about yoga workshops, retreats and training with Rachel at www.rachelzinmanyoga.com or her blog at www.yogafordiabetesblog.com.

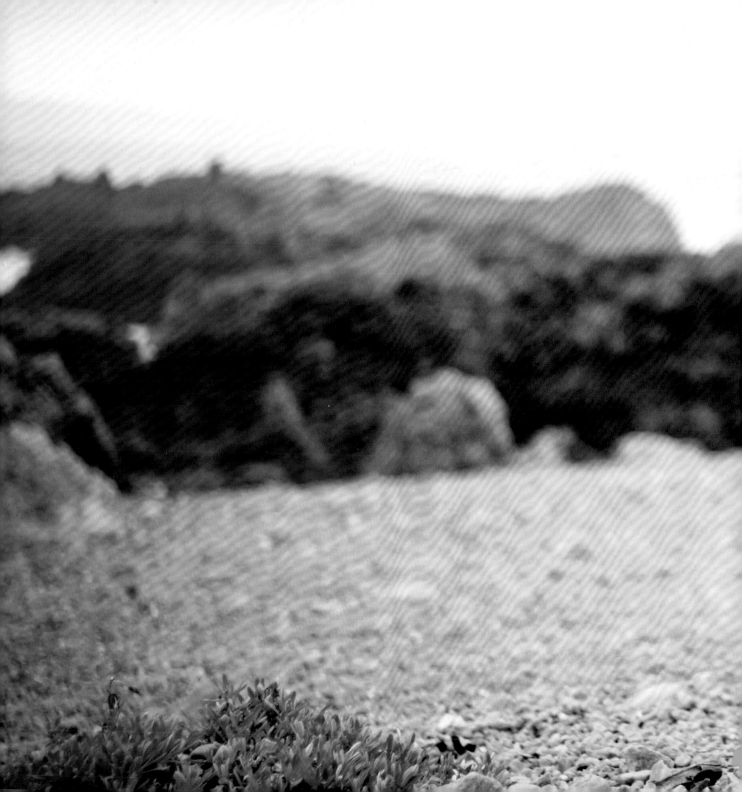

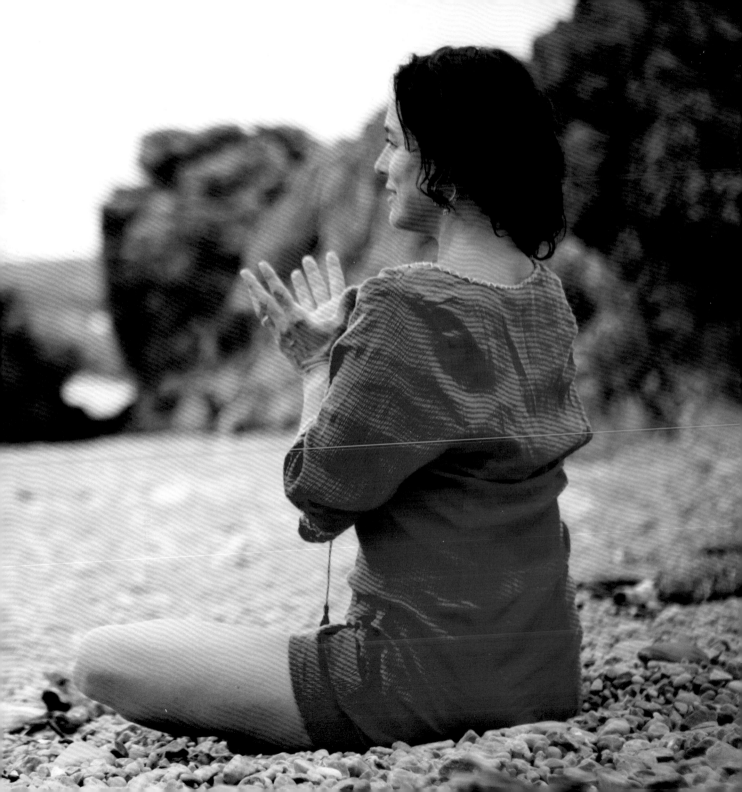